MEDICINE
in America:

A SHORT HISTORY

THE AMERICAN MOMENT
Stanley I. Kutler, Series Editor

MEDICINE
in America:
A SHORT HISTORY

James H. Cassedy

THE JOHNS HOPKINS UNIVERSITY PRESS

BALTIMORE AND LONDON

Preface and Index © 1991 The Johns Hopkins University Press
All rights reserved
Printed in the United States of America

The Johns Hopkins University Press
701 West 40th Street
Baltimore, Maryland 21211
The Johns Hopkins Press Ltd., London

The paper used in this book meeets the minimum requirements of
American National Standard for Information Sciences—Permanence of
Paper for Printed Library Materials, ANSI Z39.48-1984.

Library of Congress Cataloging-in-Publication Data

Cassedy, James H.
  Medicine in America : a short history / James Cassedy.
    p.   cm. — (The American moment)
  Includes bibliographical references and index.
  ISBN 0-8018-4207-7 (hard : alk. paper). — ISBN 0-8018-4208-5 (pbk. alk.
paper)
    1. Medicine—United States—History. I. Title. II. Series. [DNLM: 1.
  History of Medicine—United States. WZ 70 AA1 C27ma]
R151.C375   1991
610'.973—dc20
DNLM/DLC
for Library of Congress   91-7058

To Carol

CONTENTS

CHAPTER 4

PREFACE

THIS BOOK constitutes a brief introduction to the history of America's experience with health and disease, and with medicine, in its broadest sense. The work is selective rather than definitive in nature, suggestive and interpretive rather than comprehensive. In it I have dealt with medical and health-related matters during four successive stages of American history: the country's colonial infancy; its adolescence up through the Civil War; the period of conspicuous growth from then up to World War II; and, on an abbreviated scale, the post-1940 decades. I have placed the various medically related phenomena and developments in a general context of political, social, economic, industrial, and other changing historical realities. Not surprisingly, the tie-ins are numerous and complex, so much so that they can only be touched on here.

Within the chronological framework, I have focused on several broad aspects of the American medical scene. These reflect my view that health-related history is much more than the history of medical doctors and their professional concerns, important as those are. The five overriding themes that I have selected also provide continuity from one chronological section to another:

The Medical Establishment. I deal here with the so-called "orthodox" practicing physicians, their work and ideas in the mainstream of Western medicine, and their professional and institutional worlds in the American setting. I also consider allied health professionals, albeit more briefly. The book is more concerned with the collective history of these professionals than with individuals, and it treats specific institutions equally sparingly. Likewise, I have concentrated more on the general character of American contributions to medical knowledge than on individual innovations or discoveries.

Nonestablishment Health Activities. In these parts I consider self-dosage, popular health concepts, and personal choice as medical factors over the years. Particular attention is given to the successive organized movements to promote personal hygiene, nutrition, and physical exercise, and to the changing roles of the various therapeutic sects. I regard these movements and aspirations as having collectively fully as much significance in the country's medical history as those of the orthodox establishment.

The Health-Related Sciences.   The book examines briefly the characteristic individual sciences of each period, together with certain of their institutions and accomplishments. I am concerned with the failed sciences of early generations, with those that were superseded, as well as with those that prevailed and continued to flourish.

Government and Health.   I consider here the collective health needs of society in the respective periods, as well as the changing health-related responses of governments at all levels, including their involvement in such areas as health care, licensing, and research, but particularly in sanitation and public health. I treat public health primarily as an aspect of social and governmental concern rather than as a medical specialty.

Health Environments.   Here I highlight the combinations of circumstances—physical, pathological, economic, social, medical, and other—that affected the salubrity of Americans in the principal habitats that they frequented during the respective periods. My aim has been to differentiate, more than has usually been done, among the health-related quality of life of this country's rural, small town, urban, and transient populations, as well as of certain special groups.

In addition to these five principal areas of concern, I have given some attention to such matters as the ongoing tensions between the curative and preventive traditions in the United States; the differentials in health resources and services that have been available to the respective economic and social classes; the repetitive significance of war in America's health and medical development; and the close continuing ties between this country's medical ideas and practices and those of other countries. At the same time, I have omitted or given less attention to certain other topics, especially if they did not bear at all directly upon the general themes of American history or were not peculiar to the American scene in some respect or another. This has meant, among other things, giving short shrift to much of the internal (technical) history of medical practice and therapeutics, activities which have been, in kind if not in quantity, much the same in the United States as in other parts of the Western world, and details of which are readily available elsewhere.

To a considerable extent, in fact, this book is a historical inquiry into the distinctiveness of medicine and other health-related activities in the United States. In this pursuit I have tried to avoid the whiggish glorification of American medical successes, as well as the suggestion of inevitable "progress" for the better, and to suggest something of the richness and importance of medical themes in American history.

Elements of medical distinctiveness are particularly discernible in the broader aspects of American history and in its accidental circumstances. Special characteristics were implanted in American medicine, for instance, by the ingredients and timetables of American growth, by the interplay of the country's special interests and political processes, and by the exercise of the principles and obligations of American democracy. Unique health and medical arrangements have resulted from the particular connections existing in the United States among government, society, and business, as well as from the particular functioning of the nation's economic beliefs and practices. Conspicuously, during the past century, the country's traditions of free enterprise and money-making have given private medicine unusual strength and certain unique institutions. They have also effectively delayed the development of a system of state medicine comparable to those of other modern Western nations, and have made for considerable disparity in the medical care available to its citizens. At the same time, the country's peculiar circumstances of geography, resources, and climate, as well its demographic movements and configurations, have made for an unusual if not unique national outlook on health and medicine. And finally, the American medical scene has gained distinctiveness from the intangibles of the American character: from peoples' collective relationships with each other and with their environments; from their capacities of initiative and adaptation; from the collective patterns of motivation, choice, and prejudice that they imprinted on society.

I thank my colleagues in the History of Medicine Division of the National Library of Medicine, especially Young Rhee, Margaret Donovan, and John Parascandola, for their generous assistance of various kinds in the preparation of this book. I am also grateful to officials of this library for making it possible for me to devote the necessary time for research and writing and for providing substantial material support.

The finished book owes a great deal to Edward C. Atwater, John C. Burnham, Carol Clausen, and an anonymous reader for their careful scrutiny of an early version of the manuscript. I greatly appreciate their detailed, constructive, and penetrating suggestions.

MEDICINE
in America:

A SHORT HISTORY

CHAPTER 1

THE COLONIAL YEARS:
MEDICAL CONTINUITIES AND EXPEDIENTS

THE ENGLISH people setting out for Britain's North American colonies early in the seventeenth century all too often proved to have been misinformed, not only about the prospects for wealth in the New World but about the prospects for health and physical well-being. Not a few, sometimes to their eventual cost, rationalized that, as a new and relatively empty land, America could hardly fail to be more healthful than the Old World, with its long-established plagues and endemic ills. However, within a few decades it was made abundantly clear to most that the colonies, while they had their advantages, could not be considered as some El Dorado of health any more than they were the location of the reputed "fountain of youth."

In fact, many were undoubtedly deterred from making the long Atlantic trip by a foreknowledge of its manifold risks, dangers that always included potentially serious health perils. Such knowledge must have severely tested the strength of many an individual's desire for New World land, riches, or religious freedom. Moreover, those who actually ventured the trip were often subjected to the most harrowing experiences. While the resulting mortality was normally relatively small, the survivors who went ashore in America were typically exhausted, debilitated from the cumulative effects of seasickness, hunger, scurvy, and intestinal conditions, if not from severe encounters with infectious diseases.

A great many of the newcomers were thus already in poor physical condition as they began the arduous tasks required of them in the initial phases of creating their settlements. The fatigues from these labors, in varying combination with food shortages, exposure to the elements, and often severe mental depression, made the colonists even more vulnerable to fevers and other infections. Regardless of class or economic status, large numbers of persons in every colony

3

were immobilized by such ailments for long periods during these precarious early years. As a result of this widespread sickness, mortality rates tended to remain sources of intense concern for several decades. In Virginia alone, some 80 percent of those arriving between 1607 and 1625, or 4,800 out of 6,000, died of such illnesses. However, leaders ultimately began to notice the operation of what they called a "seasoning" process, under which the survivors eventually seemed to emerge with substantial immunity from subsequent onslaughts of disease. Also, to the great wonder and relief of the leaders, the mortality among the Indian tribes that lived in or near the colonies was even more disastrous than that of the whites.

After the first decades of settlement, disease experiences of the respective colonies differed in certain respects. Residents of the southern colonies, for instance, because of the region's increasing concentrations of slaves, ultimately began to encounter three formidable African diseases that were relatively seldom encountered elsewhere: yellow fever, hookworm, and the highly malignant strain of malaria, *Plasmodium falciparum*. Inhabitants of northern colonies, in turn, suffered greatly from the various illnesses associated with exposure to harsh extremes of weather. Apart from such differences, however, individuals in all of the colonies quickly found themselves facing much the same kinds and patterns of disease that they had known in the mother country: respiratory and gastrointestinal infections, childhood diseases, "fevers" of various kinds, diabetes, parasites, cancers, circulatory conditions and stroke, illnesses acute and chronic, accidents, and so on. Whatever their political, religious, or economic preoccupations, the colonists' experiences with disease and injury thus became continuing and often worrisome aspects of their lives in America just as they had been in Britain. Like their counterparts in the neighboring Spanish and French colonies, moreover, their first efforts to cope with illness relied predominantly upon measures and medications that they brought from home.

European Transfers to the Americas

Renaissance Europe's colonizing in the New World involved carrying to the selected sites such tangibles and intangibles as forms of government, social institutions, systems of belief, accumulations of knowledge, and ways of life that were then current in the Old World. At the same time, it included the transfer of Europeans' current ideas about diseases, their modes of dealing with them, their forms of medical institutions, and their kinds of medical personnel. The European states provided varying kinds and amounts of support, both initial and ongoing, for medicine and health-related pursuits in their colonies. Whatever the form or extent of this support, however, medicine in the various colonies generally took on much of the character of the medicine of the respective mother countries, a circumstance which ensured the continuance of many special transatlantic ties between them. However, many years were inevitably required before the colonies could arrive at the same level of medical quality and achievement as the European countries had.

Unknowingly, the colonization process also included the transfer of disease. The return of Columbus's sailors from the West Indies is widely credited with introducing syphilis into Europe. In exchange, the numerous ships that left Europe for the Americas carried, among other things, insidious cargoes of the Old World's infectious diseases. Contacts that ensued between the European newcomers and indigenous races from Peru to Canada thus resulted in much more than a succession of military defeats for the native Americans. The coming of the Europeans also meant the devastating implantation of measles, smallpox, mumps, and other diseases that seem to have been unknown in the Americas. The subsequent arrival of African slaves with their own special pathogens added to the process.

The Amerindian medical measures that were applied during the resulting outbreaks—herbal remedies, steam baths, religious rites—were probably no less effective than those then used by Europeans. However, lacking immunity against the new infections, the Indian populations were horribly decimated by the successive outbreaks. This rapid and often fatal spread of infections—it is now estimated that some 90 percent of the native American population was wiped out in the process—helped ensure the success of European colonial development as much as any other factor. Meanwhile, the relentless pressures, military and demographic, by the Europeans steadily drove the Indians from their lands and undermined their way of life. Surviving Indians increasingly gathered on the outskirts of colonial towns or on nearby reservations. There, white missionaries, teachers, soldiers, or physicians sometimes provided them with surgery or medical care, and in return occasionally learned about promising native remedies—the cinchona bark (containing quinine) is an outstanding example—which they subsequently adopted for their own uses. But in many of the colonies, particularly the British, the continued contacts between the two races were predominantly negative in effect. The result was a pervasive degradation of the Indians due to poverty, alcoholism, and undernourishment, together with an appalling death rate from accompanying diseases.

At the same time, the European colonies in the New World generally remained, for a considerable time, precarious toeholds of the
various tiny bands of outsiders in strange environments. The colonists' early efforts to survive not only involved them in wars with
indigenous peoples but included contending with wild animals,
harsh climates, fatigue, and hunger. And, from the beginning, provisions also had to be made for health care.

Both the Spanish and French administrations instituted far more
extensive and elaborate medical measures than did the British in their
New World colonies. The Spanish established and staffed permanent
hospitals early in the conquest period. In Mexico alone, within the
first hundred years they had built some 125 hospitals, many of them
for the Indian populations. In turn, the regulation of medical practice
and public health by official protomedicos began in Mexico City in
1525 and continued throughout the colonial period. In 1551, less than
twenty years after subduing the Incas, the Spanish created a university in Peru and began conferring medical degrees soon afterward.
In Mexico City, formal medical instruction was begun in 1579, while
nine years earlier the colony's printing press had already issued its
first substantial medical publication, the two-volume *Opera Medici-
nalis* of Francisco Bravo.

After a slow start, the tiny French settlements in the province of
Quebec were increasingly well furnished with surgeons, apothecaries, and physicians. In Quebec City, by the mid-seventeenth century
there was an appointed "king's physician" who, among other functions, presided over meetings of practitioners, inspected apothecary
practices, and examined prospective surgeons. The most important
medical institutions in the colony were the modest hospitals. Two
hospitals were established in Quebec by the 1640s and three more
later in the century, all of them staffed by nuns belonging to one or
another of the various Catholic orders. However, even with such
facilities, colonial Quebec never seems to have approached the elaborate medical organization and bureaucracy that the French later built
up in eighteenth-century Saint Domingue.

The history of colonial medical institutions, personnel, and services was frequently determined by the uncertainties of resupply
from the home countries. Tiny forts or settlements out on the periph-
ery of empire in what is now the United States were particularly
vulnerable to such uncertainties. The Spanish contingent that settled
St. Augustine, Florida, in 1565 included two surgeons and an apothecary, the latter equipped with a medicine chest, but in subsequent
years the inhabitants of this essentially military outpost often had no
one with significant medical knowledge to turn to. After 1697, small

thatched hospitals were periodically erected, with convicts, soldiers, or slaves being employed as nurses. No midwives were reported to be in the town until the 1740s, by which time a significant female population had begun to accumulate. In the Southwest, Spanish military outposts were similarly only irregularly provided with trained medical personnel, but at the missions of that area and in California the priests frequently had some medical knowledge.

Early French military outposts and settlements around the Great Lakes and in the Mississippi valley, being at considerable distances from Quebec City, were apparently little better off medically than their Spanish counterparts. However, those established along the Gulf Coast and supplied by the Company of the Indies seem to have been consistently well staffed with medical personnel and provided with fairly well-equipped hospitals. By the middle of the eighteenth century, New Orleans could boast not only its large military hospital, staffed by Ursuline nuns, but the small Charity Hospital for civilian patients, an institution that has survived up to the present.

Medicine in England's early colonies on the mainland of North America was far closer in scale and character to that of St. Augustine than of Mexico City, Lima, or Quebec. For a long portion of the colonial period it was almost totally lacking in the usual landmarks of formal medical organization and progress. Until well into the eighteenth century, in fact, no colony had more than a tiny handful of the academic or otherwise well-trained physicians around whom formal medical development in western European countries normally took place. There were almost no substantial medical publications, even of standard European works, for nearly a century after the founding of Jamestown. More striking, no colonial town had a medical society before 1736; none had an organized medical school before 1765; and none acquired a permanent general hospital before 1752.

The late appearance of these normal appurtenances of a medical establishment is not at all surprising, given the small size, provincial character, and limited resources of most of the British colonial towns. As late as 1700, even the largest, Boston, had fewer than 7,000 people. It is understandable that well-established London physicians would be reluctant to give up comfortable situations at home in favor of colonial locations that were unpromising physically and economically as well as professionally. Equally important, however, was the failure, during much of the colonial period, of medical, governmental, commercial, and religious agencies in England either to assume responsibility for the continuing supply of health care personnel and supplies to the colonies or to stimulate and support the creation of medical institutions. To be sure, the London Company in Virginia and the West India Company in New Amsterdam both originally supplied medical practitioners and even maintained hospitals for short periods. But those provisions were terminated when the colonies came under control of the British crown. While Royal governments interested themselves in matters of colonial defense, trade, and finance, they felt no obligation to build colonial hospitals or universities when even in the homeland comparable institutions were rarely given such support, at least before 1700. Moreover, since some of the colonies, particularly those in New England, proved disappointingly unproductive in the mother country's mercantilist economic design, British governments at home found little reason to pour money into them for health or welfare purposes. Royal governors accordingly were generally left to work out as best they could, with the respective legislative bodies and local leaders, their colonies' responses to such matters as epidemic threats, the sick poor, and the possible need for development of medical institutions.

This medical attitude of Britain's central governmental policymakers had a counterpart in the low opinion that ordinary seventeenth-century Englishmen held of physicians and their therapies. Those planning for long ocean trips to the colonies and for subsequent lives there were no different. They knew from hard experience that the medicine of their day, like that of their forefathers, could not be counted on to ward off the plague, cure cancer or smallpox, stay the course of tuberculosis, or do much against most of the other serious diseases they might well eventually encounter. They must have had a good idea that whether they remained in England or went to the colonies they would need Divine protection or luck as much as they needed medical intervention. And they must have noticed in the past that sick people for whom little or nothing had been done often did just as well as or better than those who had been subjected to the purging, bleeding, dosing, blistering, and other measures frequently employed by medical practitioners of that time.

Nevertheless, for all this, leaders of the organized shiploads of settlers destined to the various colonies made sure that their complements included, if not a fully trained physician, at least a person known to have some measure of medical competence. As a result, during their first few decades, virtually every colony acquired a good cross section of the different kinds of healers or medical practitioners that were then common in England and Europe. Of these, only a tiny number were gentlemen practitioners or had formal academic training. Far more often, the colonial practitioners, like the ordinary practitioners of England, came from other ranks. Conspicuous among them were the surgeons or barber-surgeons, the apothecaries, and various practitioners without academic credentials. With still less social status, but filling time-honored roles, were the midwives, together with an assortment of herb doctors, farriers (horse doctors), and other folk healers or nurses such as New Amsterdam's *Ziecken-troosters* or comforters of the sick. None of these latter types of practitioners organized themselves in America according to the traditional European guild groupings; and many or most such individuals had to supplement their medical incomes by farming or working at other occupations. Still, all continued to satisfy traditional social demands for their particular knowledge. Many of each kind gained respect as individuals, though others were manifestly incompetent if not outright quacks or pretenders to medical knowledge. In the aggregate, the wide selection of practitioners ensured the early colonists with a continuity of ordinary "British medicine," with kinds of medical care that they and their fathers and mothers had grown up with and were familiar with.

These various practitioners brought to the colonies a broad range of standard British and European medical concepts of the day. At the popular level they included a wide variety of folk health beliefs, with some based in astrology and magic. And at the more formal levels they included not only surviving strands of the ancient Galenic humoralism, but a mixed overlay of more recent ideas. These encompassed, among much else, the important innovations in anatomy by the Belgian Andreas Vesalius, in drug therapy by the Swiss chemist-physician Paracelsus, and in the understanding of the circulation of the blood by England's William Harvey.

Diseases and Medical Improvisation in the Colonial Habitat

The physical setting of this varied medical practice was also the setting for the births, sicknesses, deaths, and other vital events of peoples' everyday lives. Predominantly this meant one or another of the towns, villages, and plantations that sprang up along the Atlantic seaboard, most of them not far from the coast or from streams flowing toward it. The communities were uniformly small in scale, often unsophisticated in nature, and in many ways rural in outlook. Made up principally of farmers, seafarers, artisans, and their families, the populations of most of these towns, except for some of their leaders, had less in common with the ways of London than with the habits, concerns, and rhythms of life in England's small towns and rural manors. It is thus not surprising that the medicine practiced among them long included at least as much of the traditional therapeutic lore of rural England as it did of the intellectual concepts of urban savants. It is also not surprising, in the light of the towns' peculiar geographical and economic circumstances, that colonial efforts to cope with disease involved a considerable amount of improvisation or "making do."

Given the scarcity of substantially trained physicians, not a few of the early practitioners became itinerants to one degree or another. John Mitchell, for one, who also had interests in cartography, botany, and other aspects of natural history, during the 1740s moved around periodically from one plantation to another on Virginia's northern neck to treat the area's widely scattered population. At the same time, individuals who were not trained as physicians proved ready and willing to fill in when medical care was needed. Throughout the colonies, prominent and well-read persons who had any familiarity with medical literature often found themselves in demand to provide medical advice and treatment. In the South, these were often the plantation owners or their wives. In every colony they included magistrates and other public officials. One of the most conspicuous and able of these was John Winthrop, Jr., who made an enviable name as a healer among his constituents during his long tenure as governor of mid-seventeenth-century Connecticut.

Still more involved in the care of the sick in most areas were the clergymen. Preachers were traditionally among the best informed individuals about the vital medical events—births, diseases, accidents, and deaths—occurring in their parishes and communities. And not a few of them, from Samuel Danforth in the early seventeenth century to Ezra Stiles in the late eighteenth, and others beyond that time, kept extensive journal records of these events over long periods, often along with the various "remarkable providences" and natural phenomena long thought to offer clues as to God's will. Moreover, wherever communities lacked a physician or surgeon, preachers tended to take on medical services along with their pastoral duties. Many clergymen were well prepared to fill this dual function, one that had historical sanction as the "angelic conjunction." Some, in fact, were men whose knowledge of medical theory exceeded all but a few of the best regular physicians and whose practical medical skills must have been at or above the average of the various other kinds of practitioners. Clerical practitioners could be found in number in every colony up to the Revolution, with their ranks including such figures as Boston's Cotton Mather, New York's Samuel Megapolensis, Pennsylvania's Henry M. Muhlenberg, and various of the Church of England missionaries sent out by the Society for the Propagation of the Faith in Foreign Parts. Collectively, these preachers made a major contribution to colonial medicine, one that has yet to be fully delineated.

The frequent scarcity of medical practitioners and auxiliaries of all kinds also gave much impetus to domestic or do-it-yourself medicine. English people at home, particularly in rural areas, had always doctored themselves according to traditional practices, old family recipes, and local herbal lore before even thinking of bringing in any kind of physician or surgeon. The predominantly rural, small town, or maritime circumstances of colonial life from the beginning made for a substantial continuation of self-reliance in medical matters. In every colony, individuals and families did what they could for themselves, including taking such advice as they found in almanacs and popular handbooks, before turning to medical practitioners.

Members of a colonial family—especially the mothers, grandmothers, and aunts, but sometimes men as well—dealt with a considerable range of conditions. They made up simple lotions, syrups, and salves for assorted insect bites, burns, poison ivy cases, indigestion, coughs and colds, cuts, bruises, and sprains. They bandaged injuries, took care of the bedridden, and, with or without the aid of midwives, managed childbirths. But in serious situations they called on outside advice and help when it was available.

For town dwellers, the apothecary was an important source, both of medical advice and of medicines. Most of the latter had to be imported from England. However, there were many occasions in the early years when preferred medications were not available, particularly when supply ships from England failed to appear. There was then little choice but to turn to substitutes, namely, indigenous plant remedies. Whatever the source, the prescription of drugs was far from precise, being based principally upon the prescriber's previous experience. Mercury, particularly in its use for syphilis, and cinchona bark (containing quinine) for malarial fevers, were among the few medications that were consistently effective against given diseases. For other conditions, numerous substances and concoctions, principally of plant origin, were tried in the hope of obtaining relief. In any case, neither apothecaries nor physicians normally had the benefit of standard drug lists or pharmacopoeias until late in this period.

Within their individual limits, the various apothecaries, surgeons, and physicians who were called in by colonial families set fractures, lanced abscesses, pulled diseased teeth, gave enemas, prescribed for fevers, and sometimes attempted to relieve the symptoms of other ailments. However, they could do little for serious internal disorders, and few attempted surgery beyond minor procedures. Nor could much be done to alleviate the excruciating pain that often went with operations, as well as with childbirth. Similarly, they could exert little influence on outbreaks of such familiar and widespread conditions as typhoid, dysentery, malarial fevers, or the various childhood diseases; and they were even more helpless before the epidemics of diphtheria, scarlet fever, yellow fever, and (at least up to the 1720s when inoculation was introduced) smallpox.

In short, for most colonial inhabitants, a considerable measure of suffering from sickness and pain at one time or another was the normal expectation. Accidents happened everywhere. In certain areas some people suffered chronically from the debilitating effects of endemic fevers. In every colony, scattered individuals became insane or contracted syphilis. Everywhere, the devastating mortality among infants and young children was a particularly depressing part of the age's medical impotence. It is unlikely that the colonists were much worse off in these respects than Europeans; in fact, because the plague, which had produced the worst of the Old World pandemics, did not follow them to America, they were to some extent better off. But this could have provided little consolation.

Given the absence of real cures for so many conditions, most individuals had little to sustain them when severe disease struck other than their religious faith. Recent immigrants in every colony often did not even have a circle of friends or relatives—particularly of women—to support them in their serious sicknesses or struggles with imminent death. Depressed and alone, or with other newcomers in makeshift temporary shelters, such individuals frequently faced their ordeals without comforts, and often without nursing or medical attention for their illnesses.

As time went by and permanent homes were built, the sick person could usually be provided with at least the basic comforts and necessities. There were much more likely to be female family members around to provide ongoing care. There was also a greater chance of being visited by some kind of medical practitioner or healer, though none of these could hold out much hope of cure to the seriously ill patient. In fact, the medications administered to the sick tended to be family recipes about as often as doctors' prescriptions. Still more regular than medicine-taking in the bedside routine, moreover, and far more important in most households, were the Bible readings and other religious observances. The latter included the sick or dying person's private and often painful struggles to reconcile his life and his illness to God's plan. Equally important were the family prayers around the sick bed, together with the prayers and exhortations of the parish minister and pious neighbors.

Apart from the individual and family vigils, through the colonial period and beyond, entire communities often had no better alternative upon the onslaught of epidemics than to gather in the churches for days of organized penance or fasting. For, while civil authorities were expected to give some aid to the sick poor, no one supposed that they could do much if anything to protect the public from infectious disease. At the same time, however, the colonial towns did undertake a variety of traditional sanitary measures that aimed generally at bettering the quality of life. At an early date, small landowners frequently banded together for economic reasons to drain low-lying areas of their properties; but later on such actions were increasingly urged to improve the salubrity of the towns. Colonial officials periodically had to address themselves also to complaints connected with garbage disposal, the foul character of privies, the removal of dead animals, and the offensive odors from slaughterhouses and butcher shops. Eventually the larger towns began to pass ordinances to regulate drains and sewers, burial practices, street cleaning, food quality, wandering livestock, water supplies, and other matters. Normally, enforcement of such regulations proved to be difficult and sporadic. As a result, those of America's colonial towns that were turning into cities became progressively more filthy and unsightly, beset by a variety of stenches, and probably little if any more salubrious than their Old World counterparts. However, contemporaries often remarked that they still seemed more spacious, had wider streets and more that were paved, appeared cleaner, and had fewer poor people crowded into slum-type housing than towns in Europe did.

While routine sanitary concerns were eventually handled directly by individual town or city councils, central colonial governments not only enacted the initial enabling legislation for those activities but continued to exert at least sporadic direct controls over public health and medical matters. These initiatives were particularly conspicuous during periods of emergency, notably epidemic outbreaks. In the seventeenth century, scattered alarms of plague in western Europe and yellow fever in the Caribbean prompted the first quarantines of ships coming from affected areas. But in the eighteenth century the repeated menace of smallpox led colonial leaders to take much more extensive measures. They expanded their maritime quarantines in the various ports, sometimes established isolation hospitals (usually known as pest houses), set up barriers against the entry of the afflicted from one town into another, ordered special fumigations of houses where there had been cases of smallpox, and, after 1721, made some attempts during epidemics to segregate inoculated persons from other citizens. This accumulation of measures in certain localities such as Boston and Charleston may have had some effect upon the spread of smallpox. However, their application in the colonies as a whole was so irregular, tentative, and inconsistent that the benefit to the public health must have been negligible.

Medical Books and Sciences in the Colonies

In the public health responses of their communities, as well as in their handling of diseases as individuals, the colonials relied on well-established European practices, not all of them written down in books. However, whenever it was available, literary advice pertaining to medicine was avidly sought out. Ordinary literate individuals among the early arrivals frequently had at least a few medicinal recipes in their baggage, while learned persons—clergymen, magistrates, and judges, as well as educated physicians—often had substantial libraries covering theology, science, agriculture, and other topics, including medicine. Individuals of any means took pains to augment their collections periodically with purchases made through their London friends or agents. Even in the early years, certain libraries in some of the British colonies included not only medical works of Galen, Hippocrates, and other ancients, but examples of notable Renaissance and seventeenth-century medical writings. Then, as European learning continued its efflorescence, increasing numbers of books by such medical figures as Boerhaave, Hoffmann, Mead, Haller, Morgagni, and Linnaeus quickly made their way to America.

After 1700, the availability of British and European books improved with the appearance of booksellers in the larger towns. The supply was also slowly augmented with the gradual increase of colonial printing presses. Boston and Cambridge printers published a few broadsides, sermons, and other short works on medical topics in the late decades of the seventeenth century. While the publishing of such works, particularly medical sermons, everywhere expanded in the early eighteenth century, more strictly medical publications began to appear by mid-century, particularly reprint editions of British and European works. Actually, among the latter, few of the important theoretical or scientific medical tomes of the period were reprinted on this side of the Atlantic at that time. Rather, in response to their perception of colonial needs, the booksellers and printers confined themselves to reissuing eminently practical works such as John Oliver's advice on pregnancy; William Cadogan's essays on nursing and child management, and on gout; Thomas Short on medicinal plants; and Nicholas Culpeper's guide to diseases and therapies.

By far the largest proportion of the British and European health-related publications selected for reprinting were works not directed to physicians at all but to the layperson or general reader. There was a continuing demand for tracts on the evils of strong drink, for works on farriery and the diseases of animals, and for the accounts by Thomas Vincent and Daniel Defoe of London's plague onslaught of 1665. The greatest call, however, was for popular medical guides that would help ordinary families and individuals provide health care for themselves. One of the earliest of these, *Every Man His Own Doctor: Or, the Poor Planter's Physician,* by Virginia-born John Tennent, was reissued in the colonies more than a dozen times between 1734 and 1775. By the 1770s there were also one or more colonial editions of Tissot's *Advice to the People [on] Health,* John Hill's *Guide to Health and Long Life,* and John Theobald's *Every Man His Own Physician.* The Methodist cleric John Wesley's highly influential *Primitive Physic* was first reprinted in North America in 1764, and William Buchan's equally important *Domestic Medicine* in 1771; both had four editions during the colonial period and many more later. German-speaking immigrant groups, meanwhile, were also reprinting medical recipes and handbooks from the old country.

Equally important sources of medical information for eighteenth-century colonial Americans were the almanacs and newspapers. The content of both varied widely, from short adages dealing with popular hygiene and favorite prescriptions for particular diseases to substantial articles, either original or reprinted from British and other sources. By offering such material, the printers and booksellers provided a particularly useful service, not only to the individual citizen but, in the absence of native medical journals, to medical practitioners of various kinds. Benjamin Franklin, for one, doubtless had as great an impact on colonial health and medicine as any other individual simply through the medical material that he circulated in his newspaper and in his long series of Poor Richard almanacs, as well as through the varied medical publications issued by his press. But Franklin also contributed to medicine as a scientist, for instance through his experiments with mesmerism and the physiological effects of electricity, the creation of a flexible urinary catheter, and the development of bifocal glasses.

Other learned colonial individuals, including a number of physicians, also made occasional scientific contributions despite the difficulties inherent in their lives in the new land. In the seventeenth century, Connecticut's John Winthrop, Jr., was probably unique both in finding the time and in having the equipment to perform experiments in alchemy. Still, several other colonists in addition to Winthrop were elected to membership in the Royal Society of London, and some of them sent modest reports for the Society's *Philosophical Transactions*, particularly observations of New World biological, medical, or physical curiosities. Even more important, those who were members were enabled, through the *Transactions*, to keep abreast of contemporary scientific and medical activity in Great Britain and on the continent.

In the eighteenth century, learned men in most colonies became somewhat more involved in scientific activities of medical significance. More individuals than previously could devote time to building up their collections of natural history specimens. Some, including New York's Cadwallader Colden, Virginia's John Mitchell, the Bartrams of Pennsylvania, and Alexander Garden of South Carolina, collected medicinal and other plants, bundled packages of seeds off to European botanists, and had extended correspondence with some of them, including the noted Swedish classifier, Linnaeus. An equal or larger number of colonials had begun making regular meteorological observations, and several of these, among them Charleston's Lionel Chalmers, attempted to find correlations between weather and disease. Their published observations in the neo-Hippocratic tradition, some of book length, were regarded as important for the insights they provided into the salubrity of the New World environment.

During the late 1760s the American Philosophical Society, based in Philadelphia, emerged as one of the handful of colonial bodies devoted to the furtherance of science, medicine, and other learned fields. Of the Society's 228 American members in 1770, 42 were listed as M.D.s or "Drs." Physician-members frequently served as officers and from time to time presented papers, some of them on medical matters.

Actually, the number of original works on strictly medical topics that were published by colonial physicians, either at home or abroad, never became very large. Prominent among such contributions in the 1730s was the study of scarlet fever by the Bostonian, William Douglass. Several practitioners, including John Lining and John Mitchell, prepared valuable accounts of yellow fever. South Carolina's Lining, in the 1740s, contributed an even more significant report of his extended experiments to measure bodily excretions. And, in 1775, John Jones, then of New York, issued a treatise on the treatment of wounds and fractures, the first work on surgery to be written and published in the British colonies.

By far the most important colonial contribution to health and medicine was the introduction of inoculation against smallpox. This development occurred in America at the same time as, but independently of, its introduction in Great Britain. In both places, the decision to try inoculation was largely the result of reports, principally in the *Philosophical Transactions*, of its successful earlier use in Turkey and Africa.

In Boston, the Reverend Cotton Mather read those reports, but he had also learned about inoculation from his slave Onesimus. The highly learned Mather was a frequent writer on medical matters in a religious context. He had also lost his wife and several children from smallpox early in the eighteenth century. In 1721 he made a public plea for the trial of inoculation in the hope of controlling a new and virulent outbreak of smallpox in Boston and was able to persuade one physician, Zabdiel Boylston, to adopt the practice. Mather's vigorous public advocacy of the measure and Boylston's successful application of it on several hundred persons were quickly endorsed by most of Boston's clergymen. The remaining medical practitioners, however, led by William Douglass, the only Boston physician then with an M.D. degree, strongly opposed inoculation, partly because its uncontrolled use threatened to spread the disease. Given these differences, a vituperous newspaper and pamphlet controversy over the merits of inoculation ensued and continued through the course of the epidemic. Actually, controversy persisted until the effectiveness of the measure came to be demonstrated by experience and by statistics produced by Boylston, Mather, and others, and after controls over its use were installed. Douglass and other opponents were particularly persuaded to change their minds about inoculation after special hospitals emerged where the procedure could be administered. Use of the measure then spread steadily both in and beyond Boston. Well before the Revolution, despite certain disadvantages, it became established in most of the other colonies.

Seeds of a Native Medical Establishment

The controversy between most of Boston's medical men and its clergymen over the inoculation issue was symptomatic of a larger problem. The physicians were angry that their advice—in this case, to prohibit inoculation, at least until its safety had been demonstrated—had been rejected by the community. They were resentful as well that the contrary advice of nonphysicians, of outside "meddlers," had prevailed. The inoculation controversy came at a time when colonial physicians were not yet in a position to effectively present, let alone defend, their various perceived interests as professionals. Over the next half-century, however, their ability to do so began slowly to improve as scattered preliminary steps were taken in some of the colonies, both to achieve a measure of professional organization and to establish permanent health care institutions.

The principal factor in bringing about formal medical development in the eighteenth century was the slow but steady increase in the numbers of well-qualified general practitioners. This increase went hand in hand with such things as the general enlargement in population, the expansion of colonial towns, and the rise of a well-to-do segment of society that could command more of the amenities of life, including the best medical service. Up to mid-century, most of the sought-after practitioners were individuals who had had no formal medical education beyond their apprenticeships with preceptors. Nevertheless, with long experience many had gained solid reputations. To a limited extent, however, these practitioners gradually began to be joined by academically trained physicians. In the decades after 1700, small numbers of established British physicians, notably graduates of Leyden, Edinburgh, and Glasgow, began to move to America, where they set themselves up in practice in the larger towns. Among them were Douglass in Boston, Lining and Garden in Charleston, Colden in New York, Alexander Hamilton (not the future statesman) in Annapolis, and others. Meanwhile, by mid-century significant numbers of American-born physicians had begun to obtain formal training abroad and were returning to the colonies.

Eventually a few established physicians began offering courses in special medical subjects, principally anatomy, in the colonies themselves. After 1730 such courses were given in New York, Philadelphia, Newport, and New Brunswick, New Jersey. However, in 1765, the College of Philadelphia (later the University of Pennsylvania) established a full-scale medical school, largely on the initiative and plan of John Morgan, a young Philadelphian who had only recently graduated in medicine from Edinburgh. Two years later, Kings College in New York City (later Columbia University) followed suit. The first students at the two schools were given instruction in such standard subjects as medical theory and practice, surgery, anatomy, botany, chemistry and *materia medica* (the study of medications), midwifery, and clinical medicine. By the outbreak of the Revolution, forty-one individuals had received the M.B. or bachelor of medicine degree and seven the M.D. degree.

As the numbers of well-qualified physicians increased, they made sporadic attempts to organize the profession. One of their most desired objectives was some sort of restriction on the kinds and numbers of medical practitioners, particularly through licensing. Medical

licensing laws had been passed in seventeenth-century Massachusetts, New Jersey, and New York, but all had proved premature.
Mid-eighteenth-century medical leaders then attempted to obtain
new legislation. However, only two laws were actually enacted, that
of New York in 1760 and of New Jersey in 1772, and these also proved
unpopular and unenforceable.

In fact, the whole attempt at medical selectivity was poorly received by a considerable part of the public. Some resented the airs
often assumed by well-trained physicians, while others bridled at the
invective employed by physicians in trying to discredit unlettered
practitioners as quacks. Above all, however, many people resisted
licensure essentially because of the threat it posed to their traditional
freedom to choose from among a broad range of healers.

Much of the later colonial initiative for licensure came from newly
formed medical societies. Small groups of physicians were beginning
to meet together, at least from time to time, in some of the larger
communities by the 1730s. The Medical Society of Boston was
founded in 1736, and similar groups were formed during the next
few decades in New York, Charleston, Philadelphia, and some
smaller towns. Most, however, were short-lived. The most successful, or at least the only one to survive the American Revolution, was
the New Jersey Medical Society, established in New Brunswick in
1766. One of the early initiatives of the members of that society was
to devise a uniform fee table, but this proved to be as controversial and unworkable in pre-Revolutionary New Jersey as the licensing law.

A matter of importance to physicians both in and outside of the
societies, as well as to laypeople, was the question of hospital care
in the larger communities for those who could not obtain care at
home. Hospitals for special groups had been occasionally erected in
the British colonies in the seventeenth century, including one for new
settlers along the James River in 1612, and another for troops in New
Amsterdam in 1658. Isolation hospitals appeared soon after 1700,
inoculation hospitals by mid-century, and a hospital for the mentally
ill at Williamsburg in 1773, though only the last proved long-lasting.
Almshouses that came into being in larger towns during the eighteenth century often provided custodial and medical care for the destitute and poor with chronic illness. However, neither they nor the
special hospitals were intended to serve the strictly medical needs of
the general populace.

The Pennsylvania Hospital, which opened in Philadelphia in 1752,
did essentially this. While designed primarily for the poor, this institution also accepted paying patients. Moreover, unlike the almshouse

clientele, its patients were to be discharged as soon as they were cured or were felt to be incurable. In New York City, construction of a hospital with similar policies was begun in the early 1770s but encountered many delays and was not completed until 1791.

None of the modest professional initiatives and neither of the hospitals that were launched in the closing years of colonialism can be credited to policy changes in the British government. Royal governors, to be sure, usually lent their prestige and support to such rare ventures. But the real impetus came from local needs and energies. Up to the end of British rule, officials in the mother country played only indirect roles in the small-scale development of America's formal medicine. And they concerned themselves not at all with the unorganized therapeutic practitioners and informal health measures resorted to by the bulk of the population.

The colonial period's transfer of medicine from Great Britain to America had thus been limited mainly to the voluntary migration of individual physicians and other health-related personnel, the export of instruments and medication, and the flow of medical ideas and scientific literature at all levels. As the numbers of health care personnel grew, whether organized or not, the medical improvisation common in the early colonial period declined somewhat. Moreover, with immigration and migration tapering down to a trickle during the late colonial years, the early colonial disease crises that had been associated with the seasoning process among the newcomers also declined. This left Americans on their farms and in small-town habitats with patterns of endemic and epidemic disease which, by the 1770s, differed relatively little from those of comparable stable habitats in Great Britain and Europe.

CHAPTER 2

THE YOUNG NATION:
MEDICAL ASPIRATIONS AND
LIMITATIONS, 1776–1865

THE AMERICAN colonies that broke away from Great Britain during the 1770s and 1780s, like many a budding nation before and since, were economically feeble, politically impotent, socially and culturally underdeveloped, and far from united. In many respects, in fact, despite its leaders' efforts to devise a central structure of law and government, the United States for the next three-quarters of a century or so remained a collection of individual communities with heavily state and local outlooks, institutions, and objectives. This was eminently the case in health-related matters.

Understandably, the ordinary late-eighteenth- and early-nineteenth-century citizen's health concerns rarely went further than his or her own ailments or other purely local disease outbreaks as well as the near-at-hand sources of medical advice—family members, midwives, herbalists, apothecaries, and physicians. Likewise, the expansion of health care institutions during the period was a matter of collective local perceptions of need, while the organization of medical societies, schools, and journals came about through the initiatives of ambitious city and state practitioners. Similarly, quarantines and other responses to epidemics were the responsibilities of city and state governments. And, not least of all, the disputes that soured America's medical scene throughout this period were heavily local in nature and focus, conflicts that involved not only practitioners of every stripe and social class but often public officials and ordinary citizens as well. However, of paramount prior concern to all at this time were the even more deeply wrenching hostilities between Americans and the former mother country.

Medicine and America's Separation from Great Britain

The end of colonialism and the achievement of Independence by themselves brought relatively little immediate change in America's medicine and health-related affairs. Since the departing British had not tied the colonies' formal medical arrangements to those of the home country, there were no such mechanisms to be dismantled or replaced. At the same time, however, the paucity of certain health services proved to be a serious handicap in the Americans' extended war against the former mother country. Unfortunately this was a war that had to be fought before Americans could do much about organizing and strengthening the new nation governmentally, socially, economically, or medically.

The outbreak of war in the mid-1770s quickly affected normal medically related activity in the American community. Colonial medical students in Edinburgh and London had to cut short their studies and return home. Tory physicians packed and left, mostly for Canada or Great Britain. The ranks of the remaining patriot physicians and apothecaries, in turn, were depleted by the needs of the army, while the few health care institutions were also taken over by the military as required. The British blockade, meanwhile, quickly created serious shortages of drugs, medical instruments, and other supplies. Civilian populations suffered, but the troops suffered more.

The military medical phase of the Revolution was frequently chaotic, chronically discouraging, and sometimes calamitous to the point of threatening the whole war effort. It was dominated by desperate efforts on the part of the breakaway colonists to create a large medical organization from nothing and keep it running; to provide hospitals; to recruit and retain adequate numbers of surgeons, apothecaries, and other personnel; and to obtain critically needed drugs and other medical supplies. Within the Army, these efforts were hampered by such difficulties as severe shortages of funds, meddlings by Congress, inexperience of personnel in military matters, conflicts over authority, and vicious personal jealousies at all levels. Some of the top leaders of the medical services—in fact, the first three Directors General—were themselves causes of disruption and contributors to low morale. One, the Boston physician Benjamin Church, was removed for alleged treason; his successor, John Morgan, was removed for political reasons; while Morgan's successor, William Shippen of Philadelphia, in turn was put on trial for alleged fraud and speculation in medical supplies.

In the final analysis, however, the principal medical problems for

America's Revolutionary forces, as of any army, were the wounds and diseases. Minor battlefield injuries could often be treated, but the chances of surviving amputations were not good. Surgery was not even attempted for major chest or abdominal wounds. As in all wars up to that time, moreover, the infectious diseases that swept through the camps and hospitals could not be prevented or confined to any great extent. Control efforts were severely limited at the outset because of the minimal factual knowledge then available about disease causation and prevention. Basic sanitary measures thus were rarely insisted upon. Moreover, commanders and medical officers did not always fully utilize even such measures as inoculation. As a result, outbreaks of typhus, dysentery, smallpox, and other diseases produced devastating losses of life among the troops over the course of the war. In particular cases, the fact of these losses, such as those caused by smallpox in the first expedition against Canada, was sometimes critical in determining the outcome of entire operations.

The ending of the Revolution brought on a state of national euphoria that tended to obscure the extent of these wartime losses. It also saw the rapid dismantling of most of the wartime military-medical structure, an action which left the country about as poorly prepared medically in 1812 for a second war against Great Britain as it had been in 1775. At the same time, the coming of peace brought about a redirecting of attention to the civilian medical scene, a new focus of energies in that arena, and a general opening up of American society and the economy to the world in ways that were conducive to medical change and growth, all of these being changes that intensified after 1815.

For not a few medical practitioners, peacetime conditions permitted the restoration of some of their former medical ties with Great Britain—resumption of subscriptions to British periodicals; renewal of shipments of British medications, books, and instruments; arranging once again to send their students to British medical schools and hospitals. Equally important for some was the renewal of their personal correspondence with former teachers and professional colleagues, some of whom were such established leaders of British medicine as William Cullen, John Lettsom, and John Hunter. In addition, however, the Americans also entered into contacts with physicians of a new generation—Thomas Percival, William Withering, Edward Jenner, and others—and often with such social energizers as the prison and hospital reformer John Howard and the Tuke family, known for their innovative treatment of the mentally ill.

At the same time, postwar conditions created new channels of communication with Europe—increased links with non-British physicians and scientists, and expanded opportunities for study in European institutions. France, partly as a consequence of its wartime support of America's Revolutionary cause, offered an attractive alternative for some physicians. Jefferson and Franklin helped draw the attention of their compatriots to the late-eighteenth-century advantages of French science, medicine, and culture. Subsequently, two versatile physicians, New York's Samuel Latham Mitchill and New Hampshire's Lyman Spalding, were among those who introduced the chemical innovations of Lavoisier into the United States. Medical men on the western shores of the Atlantic became aware at an early date of such developments as the anatomical studies of Xavier Bichat and the contributions to hospital care and management of Philippe Pinel and his contemporaries. Americans, laypersons and physicians alike—Philadelphia's Benjamin Rush was one of the most prominent of the latter—were also deeply influenced by the humane strands of the French Enlightenment. These included not only its political idealism but its commitment to education and its concerns for the poor, the deaf and blind, the insane, and prisoners. However, the excesses of the French Revolution and of Napoleonic absolutism eventually turned some otherwise sympathetic American medical and reform leaders back into the British sphere. Moreover, Americans' frequent unfamiliarity with French or other languages forced many of them to continue to get their knowledge of European medical, as well as of other health-related and scientific innovations, largely through the filter of British medical literature and institutions.

Despite the various postcolonial influences from the Old World, the early-nineteenth-century growth of America's medical institutions was greatly impeded by the nation's continuing political and economic difficulties. The latter also proved to be far from conducive to the production of original contributions by medical men. This state of affairs was partly responsible in 1820 for the celebrated (and accurate) "put-down" of things American by the British pundit Sydney Smith. Writing in a rhetorical vein, Smith asked: "In the four quarters of the globe, who reads an American book? or goes to an American play? or looks at an American picture or statue? What does the world yet owe to American physicians or surgeons?" This observation had the undoubted result of rousing some to try to accelerate the slow course of American medical investigation. But most practitioners in the United States, at least the more orthodox among them, seemed to be far less concerned with making contributions to world medicine at that point in time than with trying to organize themselves in effective professional bodies.

Mainstream Medicine in a Developing Country

In post-Revolutionary America, medical practitioners were increasingly identified as belonging in one of two loose groupings. One of these was the body of "regular," or mainstream, physicians, while the second was composed of most of the others, eventually including adherents of a variety of competing medical sects. Mainstream medicine at that time was already taking on a number of features that made it recognizable to the public, distinguished it from the sects, and often made it the focus of sectarian attacks. Its practitioners, even if they had not been trained in medical schools, were often thought of as learned men, though many were not, by any means. The source of this learning, the whole corpus of Western medical knowledge, was being constantly enlarged, particularly by the experimental findings and empirical observations of European physicians. At the same time, the mainstream approach to disease and therapy was all too often based upon highly theoretical systems that had been constructed by medical savants: Friedrich Hoffmann, Herman Boerhaave, Georg Stahl, William Cullen, John Brown, and other Europeans, along with Benjamin Rush and a few other Americans.

Mainline physicians differed to some extent among themselves in their therapeutic measures, but the increasing adoption by many of them of "heroic" treatments—massive bloodletting and purging—provided the emerging sects with their most effective argument against regular medicine. At the same time the regulars were gaining in professional identity, they were also incurring increased hostility from other practitioners as well as from the general public. This was due largely to their steadily more aggressive efforts to organize themselves professionally, in effect to create an indigenous American medical establishment or monopoly.

In pursuit of their various goals, post-Revolutionary regular physicians set about once more, in one city or town after another, to establish local medical societies and other professional institutions, eventually including county and state bodies. This ongoing process, which followed the post-Revolutionary movement of population and settlement westward, paralleled the creation of educational, cultural, scientific, and other civic institutions in the various communities. And not infrequently physicians were as active in building up the latter as they were in forming strictly medical institutions. Prototypical of such individuals was the energetic and influential Daniel Drake, who was not only a pioneer medical educator in Ohio and Kentucky but a scientist with wide-ranging interests, a civic leader in great demand, and an effective publicist for the development of the West.

The steady impulse to form orthodox medical societies resulted, by the early 1870s, in over 400 such bodies. In various degrees these societies provided forums for the discussion of medical experience and scientific innovation. But above all they sought to advance the interests of the regulars and unify the rest of the medical profession around themselves. After 1808 many societies prepared codes of medical behavior and ethics, formulations that were modeled closely on the British code of Thomas Percival and which were increasingly used to draw the line between the orthodox and sectarian practitioners. Not a few of these groups also managed to prepare standard local fee tables for the various medical services, though in the face of sectarian competition these were seldom enforceable.

The societies' most significant labors, perhaps, were their renewed efforts to obtain state medical licensing laws. Considerable original success marked this effort; by 1830 thirteen states had such legislation. Yet the accomplishment was short-lived. During the next fifteen years, mainly as a result of sectarian complaints and political pressures, eleven of the states repealed their laws, while in others the provisions reverted to dead-letters. A national professional group, the American Medical Association, was founded in 1847 partly to coordinate the regulars' response to these setbacks. But it was not until after the Civil War that the regulars and their societies recovered their strength sufficiently to press successfully for new licensing laws.

Another key element in the establishment and professionalization of regular medicine was the extension of indigenous medical education. After the Revolution, the educational role of individual physicians as preceptors continued to be important, but during the nineteenth century it gradually declined as the country's medical schools became more numerous. To be sure, significant numbers of students also continued to go abroad for medical study. Not a few of them selected British institutions, but by the 1830s a considerable number had begun to take advantage of the excellent French facilities, while from the 1860s German and Austrian schools and clinics were increasingly preferred. A large proportion of those going abroad for medical study, however, was composed of individuals seeking advanced instruction.

The earliest post-Revolutionary medical schools in this country were usually sponsored by the medical societies and affiliated with existing institutions of higher learning. Soon after 1815, however, those relationships changed. Increasingly the schools began to be run virtually independently of these other institutions, tied to America's tiny colleges only by the latters' degree-granting authority. The medical schools began to act virtually as private fiefdoms of ambitious physicians, of doctors who were not only the faculty members but the proprietors of the schools. Since the organizers enjoyed the entire income from students' fees under this arrangement, the proprietary concept spread rapidly and was enthusiastically adopted as the basis for most subsequent nineteenth-century schools. Many of these, during the course of the nineteenth century, were launched on waves of "puffery," or florid promotional literature, that contemporary observers criticized as being more in keeping with business hucksterism than with scientific activity. At any rate, under the proprietary format enrollments were encouraged by virtually guaranteeing that every student would be granted a degree. And, as part of the same process, the M.D. degree for some time replaced the official license as society's main basis for judging medical competence.

Under the stimulus of the proprietary system of education, the United States, in hardly half a century, was transformed in an important way. From a land with a grave scarcity of physicians, it changed to one with more doctors than could be assimilated, at least in the country's older sections, though few of the new practitioners were more than nominally qualified. Between 1765 and 1800 the country's five earliest tiny medical schools had together produced fewer than 250 physicians. During the single decade of the 1830s, however, the orthodox schools produced an estimated 6,800 graduates, while during the 1850s the output rose to nearly 18,000.

Well before 1865, when Horace Greeley penned his famous editorial line, "Go West, Young Man, Go West," in the *New York Tribune*, medical leaders were trying to interest the large numbers of surplus young eastern doctors in medical opportunities in other sections of the country. An 1854 commentator in the *Boston Medical and Surgical Journal* put it to them in this way: "Why not strike manfully into the virgin regions of the West, and grow up with society [there], into wealth, usefulness and distinction? . . . Wherever there are human beings, there the advice of the physician is required; and as population increases, so does the odor of his good name. In short, prosperity and usefulness will in most cases be the reward of those who leave the old hive, to act their parts and gather and get gain in the unoccupied localities of Oregon, Nebraska, and Kansas."

The multiplication of orthodox practitioners and professional medical institutions was not only documented but supported, after 1797, by a rapidly increasing body of domestic medical journals organized by the regulars, the earliest of which was New York's *Medical Repository*. While small in size and frequently short-lived, the journals performed several important services. They transmitted new European information and provided outlets for local medical writers. They also attempted to promote a community of spirit among regulars. As part of this, their editors were expected to be vigorous defenders of the orthodox medical viewpoint. However, there were significant differences of opinion among the latter as to what that should be. J. V. C. Smith, editor of the *Boston Medical and Surgical Journal* between 1834 and 1856, for one, was severely criticized by some regulars for his laxity in this respect, for an alleged tendency "to shield everything except downright quackery."

Actually, at that period as in earlier and later times, mainline physicians often tended to use the term "quack" very broadly to designate and discredit virtually any competing healer, whether independent or a member of an organized medical sect. Members of the antebellum public, understandably, often rejected this orthodox usage of the word. Many of them, in fact, as well as the nonestablishment practitioners, tended just as dogmatically to regard the damaging therapies pursued by many regular physicians themselves as quackery.

For almost every variety of organized practitioner, however, as well as for the general public, there remained the problem of the actual quack—of the pretender to medical knowledge or credentials, the deliberate therapeutic fraud, the unscrupulous manufacturer and purveyor of worthless nostrums or devices that harmed rather than cured people. Such individuals became conspicuous on the American scene during the colonial period and reappeared in every later generation. Using misleading labels, they distributed hosts of questionable medications, ranging from Bateman's Pectoral Drops of the 1730s to Swaim's Panacea and Lydia Pinkham's Vegetable Compound in the late nineteenth century and others later. Entrepreneurs also merchandized huge numbers of worthless therapeutic devices, items ranging from Elisha Perkins's "metallic tractors" of the 1790s to the "Oscillotrons," "Micro-Dynameters," "Voltaic Belts," and other gadgets of the nineteenth and twentieth centuries. Given the long-lasting uncertainties of formal medicine, together with the citizenry's broad streak of gullibility, quackery planted deep roots and continued to flourish. With its potentially high profits, moreover, it proved to be hydraheaded in nature, defying the best efforts of the federal food and drug regulators of the twentieth century to stamp it out.

From the viewpoint of the medically orthodox, it was critically important to have effective individuals such as the journal editors as their spokespersons, for the professional lives of early regular physicians were all too precarious. To be sure, after 1800, clergymen rapidly gave up their earlier roles as medical practitioners and sometimes as competitors though, as if in compensation, some of them began to assume new roles as critics of regular medicine. The direct competition of the medical sects, on the other hand, became steadily more vigorous and effective. As such, it not only threatened the regular's livelihood but forced him to search his soul about the merits of his own therapies; not a few regulars actually defected to the sects. Meanwhile, the continued flourishing of presumed quacks and pretenders of many species cut into the regular's income, though this sometimes also spurred his efforts to reduce his own impotence as a healer by working for the general improvement of medicine.

For the ordinary antebellum regular physician, improvement increasingly meant carrying on a more-or-less ongoing process of trial and error on his patients with respect to the various therapeutic modes or options of the day. To be sure, not a few regulars continued to cling tenaciously to older therapeutic systems, especially those that stressed depletion of the patient through bleeding and purging. Such practitioners tended to measure their effectiveness by the amounts of blood withdrawn, drugs administered, and symptoms altered. The antebellum consumption of such drugs as calomel (mercury), rhubarb, opium, and medicinal alcohol was truly prodigious. At the same time, many physicians also took pains to build up their patients physically through tonics, stimulants, or restoratives. Most doctors also eagerly adopted quinine and other new drugs as they were introduced, and some experimented with the most effective doses of the drugs for various diseases. But they continued to be hampered by a lack of knowledge of the causes of diseases.

As the century went on, many of America's more learned physicians, under the influence of French clinicians, became progressively skeptical of the dogmatic older medical systems and their therapies. By the 1840s and 1850s, through their efforts, a decided moderation in bloodletting and in drug prescription began to be evident, particularly in eastern medical circles. Simultaneously, greater emphasis also came to be placed upon proper nutrition, careful nursing, and improved hygienic practices. And, with these measures, the aim of influencing the course of disease through active therapeutic intervention was increasingly modified by what was called "expectant therapy," accompanied by increased reliance upon the healing powers of nature.

One of the skeptics, Oliver Wendell Holmes, Sr., raised many hackles by his suggestion that almost the entire *materia medica* of the orthodox should best be thrown into the sea, where it would be "all the better for mankind, and all the worse for the fishes." Conservative believers in the virtues of calomel lotion, among others, thought that their form of medical therapy was too important a matter to jest about. But other contemporaries tended to forgive and enjoy the conceits of a physician who was also a literary figure. For most mid-nineteenth-century Americans, in fact, Holmes was far better known as essayist, poet, novelist, and catalyst of New England's literary flowering than he was as a Harvard medical professor. Over the longer run, however, his parallel careers gained added significance. With such later luminaries as S. Weir Mitchell, William Carlos Williams, and Walker Percy, Holmes was one of a tiny coterie of American physicians who gained reputations for the important contributions they made to literature as well as to medicine.

Throughout this period, the regular, like other kinds of practitioners, continued to conduct the largest part of his practice, including childbirth and surgery, in the homes of his patients. However, the slow rise of community institutions gradually took some doctors out into hospital wards, almshouses, asylums, dispensaries, prisons, and other places that sheltered groups of sick people, most of them poor.

The professional world of the early- and mid-nineteenth-century regulars was essentially white and male in its make-up. Elizabeth Blackwell and a handful of other women did receive medical degrees after 1849 and went on to organize a number of women's medical schools and hospitals. But by far their chief support during this time came from the various sects. Male regulars largely closed ranks both against the general idea of letting women out of the home and against the specific notion that women might be competent to enter the world of formal medicine. Some regulars also opposed women because they were real or potential competitors just as the irregulars and folk healers were. At the same time, however, certain regulars agreed that the admission of female practitioners could provide the solution to the acute embarrassment that often afflicted all concerned when male physicians were called in to manage Victorian Era childbirths and gynecological cases.

Antebellum black practitioners played even less of a role in organized medicine than women did. A few free blacks with medical degrees could be found practicing in the larger cities, but in nearly every case their medical education had been acquired abroad. A number of them, including James McCune Smith and Martin Delany, in addition to practicing medicine became effective leaders of the Abolition movement.

The expansion of immigration from European countries, meanwhile, brought increasing numbers of well-trained physicians to the United States. Some of these were sectarians, while others had orthodox leanings. Although members of both groups tended initially to practice principally among other immigrants, at least until they had mastered English, many were fairly quickly accepted in the professional institutions of the native practitioners.

Among the medical professionals, by far the largest number were general practitioners. However, the mid-nineteenth century began to see the emergence of occasional medical specialists. In the larger cities, some physicians began focusing on eye and ear diseases, mental illnesses, lung ailments, and other individual conditions. Superintendents of mental hospitals even founded their own society and journal as early as 1844.

Other physicians had already established practices that were predominantly surgical in nature, notwithstanding their continued general reluctance to undertake many of the highly risky and painful major operations. In cities where hospitals were erected, early-nineteenth-century American surgeons were able to develop techniques that compared well with those of European surgeons in virtually all operations then attempted. However, important innovations in fracture surgery, vascular surgery, and other types of operations were developed in physicians' private practices as often as in hospitals. Several of the most daring early-nineteenth-century surgical interventions—the gynecological operations of Ephraim McDowell and James Marion Sims—took place in small towns in Kentucky and Alabama. Moreover, the introduction of anesthesia—a breakthrough against pain that was undoubtedly America's most important medical contribution of the period—was a more or less simultaneous result of simple experimentation in several regions and in a variety of mid-century medical environments. Crawford Long contributed from his general practice in rural Georgia, Horace Wells and William Morton from their New England dental practices, and John C. Warren from his Boston surgical practice.

In what became yet another special field, male physicians had, by the 1830s, taken over much of the obstetrical practice among northern upper-class and middle-class women. However, midwives continued to have substantial clienteles among rural and immigrant women everywhere. Nursing of the sick, meanwhile, continued to be largely a function of women in the home. Hospital nurses had little status or training except in Roman Catholic institutions; in many hospitals, patients themselves performed certain of the functions of nurses. Not until the 1870s did formal schooling become an important part of nurses' training.

Two other branches of medicine, dentistry and pharmacy, were substantially organized professionally before the Civil War. Dentistry had long included more practically minded and preceptor-trained operators than formally trained individuals. In established medical circles, it was considered to be a dubious occupation with a large number of "quacks," many of them itinerants. In the 1830s and 1840s, American dentists, prominent among them Chapin A. Harris and Horace Hayden of Baltimore, initiated several steps to elevate the profession. Both an American dental text and a native dental journal appeared in 1839, while in 1840 the country's first school, the Baltimore College of Dental Surgery, was founded, together with the American Society of Dental Surgeons. Partly through these measures, along with the extensive development in the United States of new materials and techniques, American dentistry quickly set new standards of excellence for the profession everywhere. The prestige it came to enjoy in Europe by the time of the Civil War was unmatched by any other branch of American medicine for many years.

Apothecaries and pharmacists began their attempts to organize even earlier than the dentists did. An early impetus to professionalization came at a time when the vogue of heroic therapy began to make the sale of drugs increasingly profitable. Despite a movement during the Revolutionary Era to separate pharmacy from medical practice, many physicians continued to dispense medications. In this, however, they encountered progressively greater competition from independent apothecaries and druggists, as well as from itinerants and general retailers who sold drugs along with other products. By the early nineteenth century, European developments in chemistry and pharmacy made clear the need for better training of those individuals who would be compounding and dispensing drugs. This led to the establishment in the United States of separate schools of pharmacy beginning in the 1820s, along with a professional pharmaceutical journal and a number of local societies. However, national and state professional societies did not materialize until the 1850s and later, and then mainly under the impetus of well-trained German immigrant pharmacists who were refugees from the revolution of 1848.

The attempts at the professional organization of regular medicine, dentistry, and pharmacy did not mean very much to most ordinary American practitioners in these fields. Many of the matters pertaining to the medical schools were of interest mainly to the proprietors of the schools. Relatively few active practitioners regularly purchased medical books or journals in order to advance themselves professionally. As late as 1855, less than half of the regular physicians in Missouri were found to be subscribing to any medical periodical.

Meanwhile, many practitioners lived at too great a distance to be able to participate regularly in their local society affairs, while others found that the meetings they did get to were frequently sterile and not worth attending. Not a few found that internal conflicts of all sorts in the regular societies made for a chronically contentious spirit that was distasteful. The absence of certainty about disease etiology and therapy, in particular, made for continuous and often virulent controversy about the merits of the medical hypotheses that aspired to represent the true orthodox position. In the long run, however, critiques from outside the orthodox camp seemed to illuminate these matters more fully than did the squabbling within.

The Heyday of Medical Diversity

Despite their organizational efforts, the medical regulars represented only one side of nineteenth-century American health-related activity and opinion. Fully as conspicuous in the medical world, and collectively of equal significance, were the "irregulars." These were the exponents and practitioners of an assortment of hygienic beliefs, special therapies, and new medical systems that, especially after 1815, emerged as challenges to mainstream medicine for public favor. They included some concepts and practices that were far-fetched even for that day and place, but others that were as tenable at the time as any offered by the regulars. In advancing their ideas and measures, the members of this irregular therapeutic community conducted a loosely organized but effective running attack on regular medicine on grounds that it wasn't working. Asserting that the regulars did more harm than good to their patients, they brought forward horror stories of the results of heroic drugging practices and of damaging uses of instruments in surgery and childbirth. In doing so, they provided nineteenth-century American patients with some sharply delineated medical choices. Their emergence as medical competitors gradually roused the regulars, or allopaths, as they were frequently known, to conduct an increasingly purposeful and vituperative campaign of opposition to every form of unorthodox therapy. However, in that combat the irregulars gave as much as they received.

The flourishing of irregulars demonstrated that, while there was a substantial post-Revolutionary and early-nineteenth-century demand for the services of well-qualified regular physicians, especially in cases of serious illnesses, numerous citizens continued to have other preferences. Many continued to consult herb doctors or other folk practitioners, relied heavily on apothecaries for medical advice, and called upon midwives. Most people also continued to rely much of the time upon their families' accumulations of health lore and on their favorite health handbooks. In the exercise of these medical preferences, ordinary citizens became involved in the discussions over medical exclusivity, actively expressing opposition, among other things, to licensing proposals that would diminish their traditional choices of healers. These attitudes were enhanced by the developing trends toward political and social democracy and economic laissez faire. As a result, diversity remained a major aspect of nineteenth-century health-related attitudes and activity.

Egalitarian views led directly to antimonopolism in medicine as well as in commerce. They heightened popular resentments over the accumulations of wealth, privilege, and authority on the part of doctors as well as of lawyers, clergymen, or bankers. Soon after 1800, the Philadelphian Benjamin Rush could claim that medicine in the new republic had already cast off many earlier traits that he regarded as having been "royalist." Ostentatious dress and affected manners on the part of physicians had begun to disappear, "and prescriptions are no longer delivered with the pomp and authority of edicts." Samuel Latham Mitchill observed, a decade later, that America's combination of economic opportunity and democratic ideals was creating favorable conditions for an increasingly pluralistic medicine, for the appreciation of any kind of healer. And conversely, it became regarded as professional folly for physicians of any sort to criticize the "lower" classes or set themselves conspicuously above any segment of society. In fact, many people came to the conclusion that medical ideas, like others, should be routinely submitted to the democratic processes. As the New York journalist Mordecai Noah put it in the 1830s, "Our country, by its free institutions brings every question, as it ought, before the tribunal of public opinion. . . . Masonry has submitted to it—Mormonism, Agrarianism, Abolitionism, must all come to this at last, [while] medicine, like every useful science, should be thrown open to the observation and study of all."

Early-nineteenth-century Americans were often critical about these matters in part because many were perfectionists. And in this climate, the age-old ideal of living hygienically in order to ward off disease once more became a highly relevant and popular one. Having created what they thought was a perfect form of government, some tended to regard the good health and long life of the individual citizen as an attainable and worthy goal. Among the founding fathers themselves, Benjamin Rush, for one, spoke out often for such hygienic practices as sensible dressing, regular exercise and sleep, and moderation in eating and drinking. Others thought that progress toward such goals would render medical doctors of any kind increasingly superfluous. In any case, to the extent that crime, irreligion, illiteracy, poverty, idleness, immorality, and other blemishes were unacceptable to society, equally so was the neglect or misuse of the human body and mind.

America's hygienic perfectionists were motivated by domestic as well as foreign criticism of the country's bad health habits. In 1804, for instance, the novelist Charles Brockden Brown claimed that most Americans of that period passed through life without bathing more than once a year. Some thirty years later, moreover, the British writer-traveller Harriet Martineau similarly found not only that "baths are a rarity, [but that] the philosophy of personal cleanliness is not understood."

New impetus to personal health also came, by around 1830, from the updating of the classical precepts of hygiene and preventive medicine, teachings that were increasingly based on new physiological knowledge. A few of America's orthodox physicians dedicated themselves to making these concepts more prominent in regular medicine; however, most of the regulars tended to give them short shrift, if not to regard them as actually hostile to their curative efforts. As one result, the mid-nineteenth-century health reform movement tended to draw its energies predominantly from laypersons and unorthodox medical practitioners. In fact, its leadership and distinctive character came largely from such disparate innovative individuals as the temperance preacher Sylvester Graham, the physician and educator William Alcott, and New York's Fowler family, several of whom were phrenologists and publishers.

Influenced by such persons, large numbers of antebellum Americans flocked to lectures on physiology and hygiene; increased their walking and exercising; paid more attention to home ventilation and sleeping conditions; and did more bathing. Women were encouraged to abandon corsets and stays in favor of bloomers or other loose clothing. Not a few of the hygienic precepts were closely tied in with the prevailing middle-class morality. Married couples were enjoined against engaging in sexual intercourse except to perpetuate the species, while adolescents were cautioned about the alleged evils of masturbation. Meanwhile, reformers reproached all segments of the population for their scandalous excesses of eating and drinking and turned the teaching of moderation into a moral crusade.

In pursuit of health, popular books and journals on hygienic topics multiplied, public lectures flourished, and courses on physiology expanded in the schools. At the same time, some of the facets of reform became health enterprises in their own right. Invalids who could afford the expense were encouraged to travel for their health or to go for treatment to the numerous spas and health resorts. Meanwhile, Graham's pursuit of dietary improvement through his so-called Pythagorean regimen not only popularized Graham flour but led to a whole network of Grahamite boarding houses that followed his vegetarian ideas. Far larger in scale was the temperance movement, with its nationwide buildup of local societies. This was an effort that was energized primarily by the churches but one that was strongly reinforced by health reformers and medical practitioners of all stripes.

Despite the best efforts of health reformers, the ideal of a preventive medicine could go only so far. When serious illness occurred, most people insisted on curative attention of some kind. Reflecting the early American republic's emphasis on self-reliance, such attention was very frequently limited to care administered by the individual in the home. Home medication was, in fact, encouraged by a new outpouring of domestic treatment manuals, popular health literature of all kinds, and family medicine kits of various sizes. At the same time, nineteenth-century American society proved unusually hospitable to therapeutic innovations of every kind. In this spirit, both hypnosis and acupuncture were seriously tried out in limited ways during the century, and phrenology far more extensively, both by orthodox physicians and others.

Of still greater significance for the nineteenth-century American scene was the emergence of a cluster of independent medical sects. Built around distinctive therapeutic concepts, these sects appealed to a wide range of the period's grassroots prejudices and preferences, both social and medical. Explicitly antiestablishment in aim and tone, their practitioners grew rapidly in number and organized themselves to various degrees. As such they became the most conspicuous and effective competitors of the regular doctors.

Thomsonianism, a system of botanical medicine, was developed from rural folk practices around 1800 by the New England farmer, Samuel Thomson. Built on Thomson's understanding of the classical humors of the body, the system ultimately incorporated a considerable armamentarium of vegetable preparations, prominently cayenne pepper and lobelia, which were typically prescribed in large doses along with a regimen of steaming the body to cause sweating. Thomson originally disseminated his system mainly through a handbook, which explicitly encouraged readers to be their own doctors. Largely through sales of the book, the sect became immensely popular, powerful enough, in fact, to force the repeal of many of the state medical licensing laws. Extension of Thomsonianism likewise involved the creation of a number of formal mechanisms, starting with local friendly botanical societies in the early 1820s. By the mid-1830s the movement had established its first journal, *The Thomsonian Recorder*, had formed some state societies, and was meeting in annual national conventions. By the 1840s Thomsonians in some areas were even beginning to consider the possibility of forming their own medical schools. In fact, after reaching its peak as a national movement early in that decade, the sect splintered, largely over this issue of education, into a number of less potent local bodies.

Followers of another sect, hydropathy, equally resisted pressures to produce educated practitioners. In their case, they were firmly convinced that the United States, under the influence of the regulars, had already become a "doctor-ridden land," as their adherents often put it. Developed originally by the Silesian farmer Vincent Priessnitz, hydropathic therapy attracted numerous Americans as well as Europeans to the water-cure establishment in Graefenberg, Austria, during the 1830s and 1840s. Within a short time some of these individuals took the concept of "the cure" to the United States. Once established there, Priessnitz's simple approach to therapy through the intensive application of water, internally and externally, was often combined with equally strenuous preventive regimens of personal hygiene. And as it spread, its enthusiasts were persuaded that hydropathy seemed "destined not only to surpass, but to swallow up or wash away, every other medical system now existing among men."

During the immediate antebellum decades, dozens of rambling, hotel-like water-cure establishments did indeed appear around the American countryside. And, with the advent of improved public water supplies, others sprang up in the larger cities. Water-cure practitioners seldom organized societies, and the half-dozen or so medical schools that they founded during the 1850s did not prove to be long-lasting. Nevertheless, by mid-century, and for some time afterward, the water cure was the preferred therapy of a considerable segment of America's middle and upper classes, particularly women. It owed much of its success to the favorable word-of-mouth publicity of such patients, but also to the unusually effective educational role played by the *Water-Cure Journal*, an organ whose circulation made it one of the largest of America's antebellum periodicals.

A third major sect, homeopathy, contrasted sharply with both Thomsonianism and hydropathy in almost every respect except its hostility to the therapeutic excesses of the regulars. A system fashioned around the beginning of the nineteenth century by the German physician, Samuel Hahnemann, homeopathy came ready-made to the United States. A handful of American regular physicians began to embrace the system during the late 1820s and 1830s, and many more joined the sect later. However, well-trained immigrant physicians of the caliber of Constantin Hering proved to be the most effective at the beginning in spreading its distinctive concepts.

These ideas included particularly the doctrine of "like cures like," i.e., the treatment of diseases by drugs producing similar symptoms, together with the rationale of relying for cures upon extremely tiny and diluted doses of such drugs, or "infinitesimals," as they were called. Ridiculed though they were by the regulars, the homeopathic remedies nevertheless gained great popularity among Americans, particularly the middle and upper classes, because, unlike the calomel or other purgatives of heroic therapy, they clearly did no harm to the patient. At the same time, homeopaths tended to be intellectual, scientific in outlook, and placed a high valuation upon both education and professional organization. From the sect's early years in this country, Hering and other practitioners began the process of forming their own institutions: they set up homeopathic drugstores, clinics, dispensaries, and eventually, hospitals; they translated Hahnemann's *Organon der rationelle Heilkunde* and other key homeopathic works from the German; and they organized medical societies, journals, and schools. By mid-century, homeopathy was clearly the strongest of the irregular groups.

Yet another therapeutic system, eclecticism, carried the period's craving for medical options a step further than other sects did. It represented, in fact, an attempt to pick and choose from among what its adherents considered the best components of the other therapies of the day and to incorporate them in a new system. It had much in common with homeopathy, for instance, in trying to get away from heroic dosing. And it took much from Thomsonianism in relying heavily on native plant remedies. Yet its practitioners also agreed that some mainline remedies and concepts should be retained. As a sect, eclecticism, or "reform" medicine, gained special early popularity in Ohio, upper New York, and portions of New England, where its followers organized an assortment of medical schools, journals, and societies, including a national organization. Some of its antebellum medical schools gained a mixture of distinction and disrepute by admitting female students. In fact, much of the body's early energies were dissipated in vituperative disputes over this and other matters. Only after the Civil War were the controversies sufficiently settled to enable the sect to gain significantly in strength and popularity.

In addition to the four leading groups, smaller therapeutic sects also appeared periodically on the nineteenth-century medical scene. But most of them were limited in appeal and did not survive for long. Only a few of those that began around 1830, notably homeopathy and eclecticism, managed to continue effectively through the rest of the nineteenth century.

Nevertheless, during the mid-century decades most of the early therapeutic sects were just reaching a peak of influence. The emergence and often brash character of these movements represented for many Americans the fulfillment of certain deep-seated antebellum yearnings—their desire to be free from ancient authority, their rejections of special privilege, their gradual embracing of egalitarian concepts and relationships. More immediately, taken together, the sects just as much as the regular medical establishment played important roles in the period's groping search for medical certainty and improvement.

Ordinary citizens made clear their stake in this search by joining and supporting the sects in large numbers. By the 1850s, citizens of every social class were able to find alternative healers with whom they were comfortable socially and whose therapies seemed to offer them and their families something better than those of the orthodox physicians. Middle-class and upper-class patients in considerable numbers liked the careful personal attention and cautious dosing of the homeopaths as well as the hygienic discipline demanded by the hydropathic practitioners. Rural and lower-class patients in turn noticeably warmed to the simple folk therapies prescribed by Thomsonian and eclectic practitioners, but often also to those healers' own familiar rural or small-town habits, prejudices, and frequently lower fees. In addition, however, a good deal of the appeal of the sectarians may well have derived from a simple desire of citizens for medical change, along with a public perception of the deficiencies of orthodox medicine. As long as glaring therapeutic excesses marred the reputation of the latter, the ordinary citizen continued to welcome the option of turning to the sectarian healers.

A Modest Place for Science

One of the traits that, for certain of its practitioners anyway, set orthodox medicine apart from most of the sects was its base in science and the continued expansion, however slow, of its fund of knowledge through research. And indeed, far more regular physicians than irregulars were actively involved in America's antebellum health-related sciences. As such, they joined with other post-Revolutionary Americans in continuing the European scientific tradition and planting scientific institutions in the United States. While most of their activities were limited in scope, and particularly so in their effects on the outcomes of peoples' diseases, they did serve, in the aggregate, to somewhat enlarge the place of science in the hitherto all too unscientific field of medicine. In the process, scattered antebellum Americans continued to make some contributions that were of value, not only to their countrymen and women but to professional colleagues elsewhere in the Atlantic scientific community.

To be sure, no large-scale output by the sciences could be expected before the country's science teaching, laboratories, libraries, museums, and other facilities were much further advanced. The emergence of a native scientific tradition of any extent or depth also required the accumulation of wealth and the emergence of philanthropists able to support research. And it had to overcome the social stigmas that sometimes were attached to individuals who, like Boston's James Jackson, Jr., so much as suggested carrying on medical research in the midst of the antebellum period's business-oriented society.

The late-eighteenth- and nineteenth-century regular physicians who devised theoretical medical systems were not themselves necessarily antiscientific. But the systems did tend to discourage medical inquiry among those who subscribed to them. Thomas Jefferson, recognizing this in 1807, urged doctors to break away from such dogmas and to turn instead to objective observation, analysis, and experiment. American physicians took up the challenge slowly. However, by the 1830s a nucleus of well-educated medical men were engaged in observations aimed at contributing to certainty in medical knowledge and clinical practice. A few even proposed that medicine might ultimately be made as precise as the other sciences, though the majority preferred to think of their practice as an art.

In addition to some betterment in clinical observation, a number of other developments also began to contribute to improved overall medical precision during this period. Among these was the formulation of standards in pharmacy, notably the creation of a national pharmacopoeia in 1820, with procedures for updating it every ten years. At the same time, practical-minded surgeons and dentists and their tool makers became increasingly imaginative and productive in fashioning new instruments, while the discovery of new processes, such as the vulcanization of rubber, opened up other possibilities.

In turn, the gradual emergence of a native optical industry, while not diminishing Americans' demand for high-quality foreign instruments, helped make less expensive instruments more easily accessible to physicians. Microscopy, in particular, following the introduction of the achromatic lens, spread rapidly in the United States during the 1840s and 1850s on a wave of both popular and professional enthusiasm. As the capacities of microscopes improved, Oliver Wendell Holmes, Sr., remarked on the considerable temptation offered to Americans to "play instead of [work] with this charming instrument." Nevertheless, the era's operators did make fairly extensive use of the instrument in autopsies as well as in their explorations of water, food, and the parts of the body. But diagnostic or other medical use of the instrument did not become very extensive in the antebellum United States.

Meanwhile, starting even earlier in the century, medicine benefited somewhat more from an emerging nationwide interest in simple applied statistics. Doctors of almost all persuasions were swept up in a craze for quantification. While the results were mostly crude by later standards, the applications proved increasingly useful, not only in the administration of medical institutions and in summarizing research observations but in bolstering the claims of the respective sects.

In other respects, the early American medical institutions often seemed to have little to do with science. Still, the professional societies did provide opportunities for physicians to talk among themselves about the scientific aspects of their profession. The hospitals and asylums, for their part, offered enlarged opportunities for the observation and study of various illnesses. Meanwhile, until at least the 1840s, medical schools served effectively as one of the country's principal sources of education in the sciences; some students enrolled in them primarily in order to obtain such training and then went on to pursue nonmedical careers. At the same time, however, the rush of students to medical schools greatly stimulated the writing or translation of textbooks for the various courses. Although the practical exposure to science provided by those courses was often only elementary, the texts themselves tended to reflect Americans' steady absorption of Europe's growing knowledge and techniques in the respective sciences.

Anatomy, for one, rapidly became more complex during this period. In the United States as elsewhere, the teaching of anatomy had long relied to a large extent upon the dissection of cadavers. All too often, however, cadavers were in short supply. In such instances, grave-robbing was often resorted to, sometimes by the students themselves but sometimes by paid resurrectionists. In both cases the practice became a source of bitter community hostility against the medical schools, with the violent details of New York's "Doctors' Riot" of 1788 being periodically reenacted elsewhere throughout the antebellum period. Almost invariably, these incidents grew out of a generalized resentment of medical authority on the part of a segment of the public in combination with immediate hostilities prompted by the violation of the remains of family members or friends.

After 1800, the interests of many physicians turned to morbid anatomy, or pathology. In the pursuit of pathology, the practice of making postmortem examinations spread rapidly, though that practice also sometimes had adverse community repercussions. Such examinations, among other uses, had extensive practical applications, such as providing evidence for coroners and criminal courts. They also proved invaluable in applied research aimed at sorting out the differences among several of the period's common infectious diseases. Under the influence of pioneers in the French hospitals, a small band of antebellum physicians—Henry I. Bowditch, William Gerhard, George C. Shattuck, and others—introduced the simple but laborious "numerical method" of quantification into American clinical medicine, particularly in diagnosis. For these few investigators, at least, the century's Protestant work ethic found a place in the pursuit of medical improvement.

Meanwhile, at least some Americans around 1840 began following and duplicating the work of European investigators in such special fields as histology, embryology, and cellular pathology. However, it was not until after the Civil War that individuals trained in German laboratories were in a position to contribute materially in such areas.

In physiology, William Beaumont, an Army surgeon stationed at a small frontier post, made a distinctive and much admired antebellum contribution. This consisted of his observations of the digestive processes, thanks to the unhealed wound of a French-Canadian trapper. Apart from this, substantial studies in the field were few in the United States until after Americans had familiarized themselves with European experimental methods. Claude Bernard's demonstrations in Paris began attracting Americans in the 1840s and eventually influenced the work of such physicians as the New Yorkers John Call Dalton, and Austin Flint, Jr., and S. Weir Mitchell of Philadelphia. After 1865, however, it was Carl Ludwig's laboratory in Leipzig that increasingly attracted Americans for advanced training in physiology. As one by-product, it also provided Henry P. Bowditch with the model for America's first physiological laboratory, established in 1871 at the Harvard Medical School.

Among late-eighteenth- and nineteenth-century American physicians and intellectuals, few scientific matters were of more concern than those pertaining to "race." Some, especially in the South, interested themselves in the nature and distribution of diseases among the blacks. But other scientific questions pertaining to blacks stirred up greater interest as well as some research. Among these were questions of skin color, of acclimatization, and of whether the Negroid race had descended from a common ancestor of the other races or was a separate species. While the latter question was discussed principally within the context of Biblical authority, the argument for separate creation was considerably reinforced by the rise of craniometry and phrenology.

Phrenology, the classification and study of mental faculties through measurements of the skull, came to this country in the 1820s. It had a considerable vogue not only among the public but also, until it was taken over by itinerants and showmen, among orthodox medical practitioners. Eminent physicians, in fact, with specimens acquired from all over the world, built up some of the country's largest collections of skulls. And several—notably Samuel Morton, in Philadelphia, but also Charles Caldwell and Josiah Nott—went on to utilize the collections, both in instrumental measurements of brain size and in other comparative studies of the various human races in the tradition of such European investigators as Johann Friedrich Blumenbach and James Cowles Prichard.

Along with their ethnological activities, physicians played active roles in the ongoing exploration of the New World environment. In every state and territory, medical men were prominent among those who combed the countryside for new plant species, studied them, shipped samples off to European naturalists, and added some to the *materia medica*, the medicines in active use. Some, including the physician-botanists Benjamin Barton of Philadelphia, Jacob Bigelow of Boston, and John Shecut of Charleston, as early as 1800 began cataloging native medicinal plants according to the Linnean or other classifications and preparing elaborate publications of their work.

Other physicians collected data on the geological and topographical makeup of local environments, while large numbers made regular readings of temperature, humidity, and rainfall. The more systematic observers among the latter played significant roles in helping to put applied meteorology on an organized nationwide basis before the Civil War. Certain early- and mid-nineteenth-century medical men, moreover, examined such data along with their case records and the official bills of mortality in hopes of shedding light on the presumed close relations between environmental phenomena and disease. The St. Louis naturalist-physician George Engelmann, for one, wanting in 1853 to test common folk beliefs about such relationships, made a simple comparison of the diseases he had treated over a seventeen-year period with the the weather data that he recorded during the same time. A number of popular maxims seemed to be substantiated:

A wet summer is a healthy summer.
A wet fall is a healthy fall.
A dry and hot summer is a sickly summer.
A dry fall, whether warm or cool, is a sickly fall.
A wet summer and dry fall combined make the most sickly fall.

On a much larger scale, during the 1840s and 1850s, a few investigators, particularly Daniel Drake, Mobile's Josiah Nott, and the Army surgeon Samuel Forry, carried out pioneering studies of some of the broader physical settings and patterns of disease in the United States. And, working from the same environmental premises, still other investigators began conducting systematic surveys to pinpoint local circumstances and distributions of disease. In fact, environmental and epidemiological inquiries of these types were among the earliest medical investigations to be undertaken in nearly every region of the country. As such, they represented one phase of the gradual spread of the scientific tradition and method. But they were also expressions of peoples' very personal concerns for the salubrity and quality of life of the communities in which they lived.

Salubrity and Illness: The Nation and Rural Habitats

Most individuals continued to look at health matters in far more subjective ways than the environmental investigators did. In fact, after the Revolution, Americans as a group tended to assume that their new republic was a more salubrious place to live in than the Old World, with its presumedly corrupt monarchies and institutions. Moreover, it was generally accepted as a truism that the American countryside with its free yeoman farmers was healthier than the towns and cities. However, people's actual experiences with disease frequently cast doubts on such broad assumptions. At the same time, the collective impact of illness stimulated communities to provide ever more numerous curative and preventive institutions as the populations' needs expanded.

In general, nineteenth-century white Americans probably did not perceive disease much differently than their European contemporaries did. But, given their particular social and environmental circumstances, their experiences with it sometimes differed. Many continued to be fatalistic about disease, to view it, especially in its extreme manifestations, as an evidence of God's will. But people increasingly saw illness as something that society and the medical profession, aided by the hygienic discipline of the individual, ought to be able to alleviate or prevent, even if the actual capacity to cure all too often remained elusive.

These kinds of changing perceptions and expectations were concentrated, above all, at the bedsides of the age's seriously ill and dying. Among poor migrants, immigrants, and other transients, as well as among other poor persons, the scene at the sickbed was often a repetition of the group sicknesses of the colonial era. Large numbers of individuals in these traveling groups were likely to be homesick, hungry, fatigued, and depressed to some degree in their strange and comfortless new circumstances, with the well among them frequently little better off than the badly ill. Moreover, their numbers were generally so large that charitable and medical assistance for them in cities and towns along the travel routes often could not be obtained. In Cincinnati, New Orleans, and other Mississippi Valley communities during the 1820s, the itinerant preacher Timothy Flint came across "multitudes" of these sick and helpless transients huddling in miserable hovels, friendless, without money for food or medications, and many dying "unnoticed and unrecorded," even by local clergymen.

Among better-off classes, the ill at least had relatively comfortable circumstances for their suffering. Ongoing nursing and other care was generally supplied by family members, with frequent help from neighbors. In the course of the early nineteenth century, as they became more conscious of hygienic matters, family attendants tended to keep the sickbed environment cleaner and better ventilated, with more frequent changes of bedsheets and bathing of the patient. When physicians were brought in, it was often with great reluctance on everyone's part, though these attitudes depended much on the physician's reputation or therapeutic persuasion. The coming of the surgeon, of course, invoked the most intense fears and apprehensions on the part of the patient and the family. Calls by the old-line regular doctor, in turn, as well as by the Thomsonian healer, were likely to be almost equally feared since they were known to often consist of highly strenuous attacks on the patient's ill body, with therapies that tended to leave the patient exhausted if not also suffering from damaging side effects. The homeopath or the new-line regular physicians, on the other hand, with their generally more moderate therapies, tended to be met at the sickbed with little fear.

Families of the seriously ill, meanwhile, as well as the patients themselves, continued to rely heavily on their personal religious faith to help them through the painful and sometimes protracted periods of illness. Regular family devotions were supplemented by special prayers, while visits from the minister and members of the family church were essential elements in bolstering the patient's spirits and

resolve. During the early decades of the nineteenth century, clergymen and mainline physicians habitually collaborated closely in their
attentions to the sick. By mid-century, however, relations between
the two professions had soured in some respects; in certain communities, physicians even tried to bar the clergy from the sickroom. At
the same time, many physicians were still so lacking in confidence
in their therapies that, like the clergy and patients, they continued
to see the outcome of disease—cure or death—as a matter of God's
will. However, with the passage of time, patients came to expect
steadily more from medical science. They and their families thus were
more likely than ever to change doctors than to change ministers
when neither proved effective against painful and fearsome diseases.

For the general public, meanwhile, the farthest-reaching and most
terrifying disease manifestations were the periodic epidemic outbreaks. Most such diseases were feared at least partly because of the
continuing lack of knowledge about their causes and modes of
spread. By mid-century, Philadelphia's John Kearsley Mitchell, together with Josiah Nott, John Riddell of New Orleans, and a few
others had begun, on still unclear evidence, to blame such diseases
on microscopic animalcules or germs. But for most physicians, the
weight of evidence seemed to implicate instead such factors as
weather or topographic conditions, the decaying of local organic matter, or miasmata from other sources. Except for smallpox and, late in
the period, some of the filth diseases, there was wide continuing
uncertainty about how to prevent or control the great epidemics.

Typhus and typhoid thus occurred in epidemic form too often
during this period wherever the poor, construction gangs, prisoners,
or other groups were thrown together in numbers. Diphtheria and
other childhood diseases increased in virulence as the nineteenth
century went on. Smallpox continued to return in damaging outbreaks throughout the century and beyond, particularly among frontier populations and Indian tribes. But in much of the country its
impact was greatly reduced following the rapid introduction of vaccination after 1800. Perhaps even more feared was yellow fever. Epidemics of this disease had ravaged Atlantic port cities periodically
through the eighteenth century as far north as New England and
reached a high point in a series of particularly destructive and disruptive onslaughts between 1793 and 1820. It then retreated into the
South, which suffered periodic highly devastating visitations through
much of the rest of the century. In addition to this dreaded disease,
between 1832 and 1866, the entire country also suffered through three
massive incursions of the equally feared Asiatic cholera, each of
which brought great loss of life. The threat of additional attacks of

this disease remained as a fearful possibility for Americans throughout the remainder of the century.

Colossal as the various epidemics were as causes of death, illness, and social disruption, they nevertheless remained episodic afflictions rather than constants. In fact, various nonepidemic diseases, while less spectacular, in the aggregate, decade after decade, resulted in far more suffering, death, and grief. Cancers, cardiac conditions, and other diseases of internal organs were prominent among those ailments for which little could be done beyond sometimes relieving the symptoms. In the South, hookworm infestation and pellagra became progressively more deeply entrenched as a debilitating incubus of endemic illness among an impoverished rural population, while malarial fevers were equally deep-seated there and in the Midwest. Everywhere, tuberculosis remained the biggest single killer, particularly among adults, while dysenteries and poorly differentiated fevers continued to be dangerous facts of life. Gastrointestinal ailments and fevers, in fact, along with the various childhood diseases, kept infant mortality at an appalling level, albeit one that people were often fatalistic about. The loss of mothers in childbirth, while not quite as calamitous, remained high; few women benefited as yet from mid-century studies by Oliver Wendell Holmes, Sr., and the Hungarian Ignac Semmelweiss, which concluded that physicians themselves were the agents in the spread of much of the puerperal infection from one mother to another.

Regular medical practitioners of the period were also laid open to criticism by the physical damage that their heroic therapies often did to patients and by increases in addiction brought about by their prescriptions of opium as a medication. Patients themselves, of course, had to bear the responsibility for the incidence of diseases resulting from alcohol abuse and overeating, sometimes for venereal disease, and often for excessive self-dosing.

Meanwhile, the mentally ill, many of them newly transferred from the country's jails and garrets to hospitals during this period, were being increasingly recognized as making up one of America's largest categories of sick people. Early antebellum physicians often attributed mental illnesses to religious enthusiasm, sexual excesses, disappointed love, or business stress. But increasing professionalization in this area of medicine, along with more intensive observation of cases, was beginning to bring about somewhat greater precision in diagnosis and understanding of such illnesses.

Nineteenth-century laymen as well as medical practitioners were sometimes involved in the process of sorting out the diseases and assigning more precise names to them. They also participated in attempts to learn the quantity and distribution of deaths due to the various disease conditions. Almost none of the registration mechanisms that were adopted, official or otherwise, came close during this time to obtaining complete and accurate vital data for any segment of society. But the statistics did begin to reflect much about human life and death in the principal American habitats. Equally important, they provided increasingly rational bases for deciding where and when health care institutions should be erected.

America's medical and health profile during the post-Revolutionary and antebellum periods was anything but uniform from one decade to another, as well as from one section to another. For one thing, having been settled at different times, the various areas proceeded to grow on different demographic and developmental timetables. Medically as well as socially, culturally, governmentally, economically, and in other respects, the Northeast and eastern seaboard areas generally remained ahead of other areas simply because they had started earlier. In turn, deep southern, midwestern, and far western states or territories lagged to varying extents, depending on the influx of population and creation of basic institutions. At the same time, while the multiplication of professional medical bodies as well as of formal health care and preventive institutions was predominantly an urban phenomenon, throughout virtually all of this period the cities collectively were the habitats of only a minority of the nation's people. The majority was distributed among a number of other habitats that differed significantly from each other in their health experiences and medical arrangements, primarily the transient community, the farm, and the small town. The remembered lore of such experiences in these three habitats, in fact, furnished subsequent generations of Americans with some of their most durable images of the quality of life in the pioneering years of the United States. But in many cases, the harshnesses of the experiences were lost from the images that were retained.

With the opening up of the vast interior of the continent, transience became an increasingly conspicuous aspect of post-Revolutionary and antebellum American life. Quite apart from short-term travelers, immense numbers of people were in motion. Some had no permanent base, while others had nominal family roots but remained away from them for long periods of time. Among the transients were migrants going from one section to another; immigrants spreading out over the land; explorers and surveyors of the national resources; adventurers and hoboes; frontier troops, hunters and loggers; seekers of health, wealth, or cheap land; itinerant artists, healers, drummers, and clergymen; laborers on turnpikes, canals, and railroads; fishermen and mariners at sea.

The health environment of the transients was as varied as their modes of conveyance, and as mixed as the tents, shacks, or hotel rooms, if any, that they actually slept in. For those who enjoyed strong constitutions and optimistic temperaments, who were well provided with necessities, and were lucky, the process of going out into the vast country could be and frequently was carefree and exhilarating. Such individuals often had less sickness than they had had in previous habitats. And their often upbeat accounts of their experiences tended to obscure or downplay the frequent harshness and illness of the transient life.

Many others discovered, for instance, that infectious diseases often spread dangerously among bands of travelers. Malarial fevers took large tolls wherever immigrants had to cross swampy lands. Careless hygienic facilities and practices among all kinds of transients ensured much diarrhea, dysentery, and sometimes typhoid or typhus. Meanwhile, the poverty of many such individuals left them poorly clothed, undernourished, and inadequately protected from exposure to harsh elements. All travelers, even the relatively well-off, were subjected to frequent fatigue and to accidents. Many were lonely, homesick, or fearful; Timothy Flint and others particularly remarked on the waves of depression that swept over many an immigrant and migrant group.

While the transient habitat fostered more than its share of ill health, its resources for dealing with disease and caring for the sick were far less than those of any other habitat. Well-to-do and organized emigrant groups crossing the prairies, as well as Army exploring expeditions and merchant ships on long voyages, sometimes included physicians. But most individuals and families, except when they went through an occasional town or came to a military post, had no resources but their own. For them, medical self-help was not an ideal but a necessity. Old family recipes and travelers' medical handbooks were their primary health guides, while the supply of medications was limited to whatever they brought in their kits or discovered from among local plants. By the 1830s and 1840s, all who could afford it at least made certain to have with them a supply of Sappington's pills, a popular form of quinine that was widely credited with making the westward movement a healthier phenomenon.

Another medical aspect of this constantly moving habitat was the spread of diseases from the travelers to peoples encountered along the way. The explosive dissemination of cholera in towns and plantations along the immigrant routes between 1831 and 1866, and even into California with the gold seekers of 1849, was a particularly well-advertised instance of the phenomenon. But other moving groups were often as lethal in their impact as the immigrants were.

Particularly devastating was the continuing harvest of disease and death resulting from the relentless demographic pressures of whites in general upon the native American Indian populations in all sections of the country, which greatly intensified in the late eighteenth and nineteenth centuries. The whites' relentless grab for land forced one Indian tribe after another out of its ancestral lands, with a calamitous resulting decline in the Indians' fortunes and population. Some of the Indians were killed in battle, while many others died of hunger, from the effects of alcoholism, or of the hardships of forced removal to reservations. The artist George Catlin concluded in the 1830s that "the sword, the bayonet, and whiskey" were the most conspicuous causes of the Indian decline. But many of his contemporaries agreed that infectious diseases were by far the greatest killers. Whether these happened to be whooping cough, measles, or some other malady, and worst of all, smallpox, the Indians' contacts with the advancing whites and blacks meant exposure to pathogenic organisms against which the Indian populations had little developed immunity. By the Civil War, the tragic process had reduced those populations to only a tiny proportion of their former numbers.

The hygienic and medical environment of the farm, while similar in some respects to that of the transient community, had its own patterns. Farm life was shaped by an even more complex symbiosis with the seasons and weather, the forests and swamps, the animal life. If the farm family obtained fertile land, stayed in good health, and had continued good fortune, it could hope to enjoy the best fruits of the American dream. But the farm as habitat was notoriously vulnerable to outside forces—to drought and flood, to the ravages of insects, to distant market whims and other economic changes, and eventually to government interventions. At the same time, virtually everything accomplished was dependent upon the family's own energies and continued good health—the clearing, cultivation and draining of land; the growing of crops; tending the stock and doing domestic chores; the maintenance of barns, house, and equipment.

Healthwise, for many new settlers starting their farms in rural nineteenth-century America, just as during the colonial period, the worst part often came during the first few months. This was the stage known as "seasoning," a time when the exhausting early labors and privations left the settlers more than normally vulnerable to various infections and debilitating fevers. At every stage, the isolation, risks, and failures of continued farm life did much to enhance tendencies to mental depressions; the "lives of quiet desperation" that the writer Henry Thoreau found among his rural Massachusetts neighbors in the 1840s were replicated in the back country everywhere across the United States. The remoteness of farms from helpful neighbors, mid-wives, and medical practitioners also made childbirth of any complexity potentially dangerous, both to mothers and infants. Opportunities for accidents on the farm were legion, and they swelled during the century with the introduction of new farm machinery. Outbreaks of infectious diseases were disruptive even when there were no deaths. The springs or wells that furnished drinking water might or might not be clean, while privies and barns were typically malodorous, offensive, and capable of spreading infections. Finally, endlessly exasperating and sometimes worse were the bites of insects and the frequent poisoning from various plants and berries.

Health care was almost as much a matter of self-reliance for the farmer as for the traveler. However, most farms had a somewhat more extensive supply of medications and instruments, as well as a better chance of replenishing them when they ran out. There was also shelf room for a variety of medical handbooks. Do-it-yourself veterinary medical manuals were about as important on the farm as those for human illnesses. Not infrequently extended families provided a core of mutual support and care during severe illnesses or childbirth. While rural roads remained wretched up into the twentieth century, many farm families were close enough to a village to be able to summon a physician in an emergency. But, for lesser problems, it was often a matter of turning to the services and therapies offered by the varied itinerants who turned up from time to time— patent medicine salesmen, tooth pullers, blood-letters, bone-setters, and assorted healers.

Southern plantations, as particular kinds of farms, had their own special health circumstances. On the plantations, the predominantly black populations were subject to nearly all of the diseases of whites. However, their effectiveness as laborers in the hot southern climate was immensely enhanced by the fact that many of them enjoyed some genetic immunity to yellow fever and to certain strains of malaria. At the same time, the mortality among the young children of slaves was far higher than among white children; modern scholars agree with the planter Thomas Affleck that the ratio was approximately "as two to one." Antebellum whites also noted that the slaves as a whole suffered greatly from respiratory diseases, were often infested with parasites, and were considerably more subject than whites to rheumatism, diseases of women, urinary problems, and tooth decay. One southern physician, the controversial Samuel Cart-wright, in addition alleged that the blacks were peculiarly prone to social diseases to which he gave such names as "drapetomania, the disease causing slaves to run away," and "dysaesthesia Aethiopis," or rascality.

Health care measures on the plantations were varied. On many plantations, slaves using African folk-healing practices cared for other blacks, while black midwives were common. At the same time, how-ever, the plantation owner, his wife, and/or overseer were normally involved in providing medical care to the slaves. They frequently administered medications and performed such operations as tooth removal, bleeding, and purging. They also made arrangements with physicians in neighboring towns to visit the plantations regularly or to be on call in the event of serious illnesses or accidents. Larger plantations even maintained infirmaries. On the other hand, few owners seem to have done much about such matters as the drainage, ventilation, or sanitation of slave quarters. Moreover, the food that they provided to the slaves, while ample, seems to have rarely been on a par nutritionally even with the institutional fare of the day.

Under this combination of circumstances the slave population of the antebellum South somehow managed to show a steady natural increase, something that could not be claimed for the free blacks of either southern or northern cities. Southern apologists for the "pecu-liar institution," including many physicians, naturally made much of these figures as the century went on. However, among northern abolitionists there was little doubt that the overall health environment of the plantations was decidedly unfavorable, particularly when they considered the demoralizing and crippling effects of bondage upon the slaves.

The distinctive health environment of the third major rural habi-tat, the small town, was shaped primarily by the greater aggregations of people over those of most farms. On the one hand, of course, social togetherness in the towns multiplied both the chances of con-tracting infectious disease and the problems arising from poor sani-tary practices. On the other hand, it was beneficial in eliminating much of the isolation of farm life and in providing an enlarged sup-port network of individuals to call upon when in ill-health. Malaria was often reduced by the cooperative draining of swamps, while the general quality of life was enhanced by products and services avail-able from town merchants.

Since small-town inhabitants almost invariably continued to live as families in separate dwellings, they were each largely responsible for the environmental conditions affecting their own salubrity. This meant providing for the disposition of garbage and trash and ensuring the cleanliness of their own wells, kitchen drains, stables, and outhouses. The overall sanitary quality of American small towns thus varied widely from place to place, though many improved in this respect during the nineteenth century. Nineteenth-century town residents in any case had to have considerable tolerance for ordinary odors, those from manure piles if nothing else, and sometimes those from butcher shops and other trades. When the nuisances became too offensive it was generally hoped that community pressures or ordinances would bring relief.

In the small town as in other habitats, the family continued to depend very heavily upon its own resources for medical care. But there were also varied medical professions and resources near at hand that could be turned to. Small-town physicians, whether orthodox or irregular, were normally general practitioners who treated the sick and performed operations in the patients' homes. Many communities also had dentists and veterinary practitioners. Some towns had separate drugstores, but patent medicines and medical supplies were widely sold in general stores as well. Midwives and other female attendants generally were available to assist in deliveries or to nurse the sick or elderly. Small towns also tended to be attractive to itinerant healers of every description. However, few villages or towns had any sort of hospital or clinical facility through this period, though many counties were beginning to establish poor farms or "old folks" homes.

Health and Disease in the Growing Urban Habitat

The fourth major post-Revolutionary habitat, the city, originally had a good many hygienic similarities to the small town. But these disappeared rapidly as the cities grew larger. Colonial Americans, with only their handful of tiny cities, had long tended to think of the large European cities not only as seats of crime, immorality, and extravagant living, but as centers of disease. Nevertheless, following the Revolution, increasing numbers of people moved from America's farms and villages into its cities. There they tended to live in different types of dwellings than before, changed to new and frequently more sedentary kinds of occupations, and began to experience new patterns of health and illness, particularly as they were joined by ever larger numbers of new immigrants.

The health environment of the cities became steadily more complex as the populations grew. In particular, the residential areas tended to divide into several distinct environments, largely according to social class and financial status. The conspicuously well-to-do typically clustered in areas of spacious homes, often with stables, other outhouses, and large gardens in back. They normally had servants to prepare meals and perform household chores, including refuse removal and routine home sanitation. The neighborhoods of the wealthy frequently had quiet and shaded streets, and sometimes had river views and were within easy access to parks or, by the 1840s, scenic "rural" cemeteries. The inhabitants were clearly able to afford the best physicians and specialists as well as trips to spas or resorts for their health.

At the other extreme, the poorest inhabitants were increasingly forced into cramped tenements or hovels along the alleys of the city or near the rising factories. There they lived with only the barest of necessities, with few sanitary facilities, and in chronically poor health. Few could afford enough food or clothing, let alone patent medicines, and the only formal medical care they received was the frequently hasty if not begrudging attention given to charity patients.

In between the rich and the poor, those who belonged to the upper middle class enjoyed many of the health advantages of the wealthy. A growing lower middle class, however, one composed of the families of tradesmen, clerks, and mechanics, along with widows and others, lived in yet another environment. These were people who usually ate regularly, sometimes went on outings to the public parks, and somehow managed to buy medicines and pay doctors' bills when they became necessary. Their apartments or houses were modest and generally clean, but their efforts to dispose of household wastes—sewage, garbage, drainwater—became increasingly frustrated. Meanwhile, the streets they lived on were all too frequently noisy, congested, and piled with trash and animal manure, while the open public drains that carried off wastes were foul in the extreme. On the balance, the quality of life for much of this lower middle class throughout the period often tended to be closer to that of the poor than to that of the well-to-do.

For the populace in general, in fact, though boards of trade and newspapers persisted in claiming the reverse, nineteenth-century American cities, particularly in the North, rapidly lost a large part of whatever salubrity and pleasantness they had enjoyed as small towns. Odors from rendering firms, factories, privies, decaying garbage, and animal wastes were increasingly intense and nauseating. The use of coal after the early decades of the century, particularly in factories and railroads but also in homes, produced a pall of smoke that left deposits of soot on clothing and in houses, and increased the incidence of respiratory diseases. The basic activities of commerce, including the construction of urban buildings, streets, and public works, ensured a continuous harvest of accidents of all kinds. Moreover, the hectic pace of business in itself was presumed to produce tensions and mental breakdowns. Both the New York preacher Henry Ward Beecher and the Hartford psychiatrist Amariah Brigham, among others, saw this as a serious and widespread phenomenon.

Yet another crucial factor in the declining hygienic quality of nineteenth-century urban life, as well as in the overtaxing of housing, basic sanitary arrangements, and other civic services and institutions, was the great influx of population. Drastic overcrowding of the newcomers greatly enhanced the opportunities for the exchange of diseases of all kinds. But particularly worrisome, given the adverse environmental circumstances, was the likelihood of damaging increases of the so-called filth diseases comparable to those that had overrun European cities a generation or so earlier.

The responses of American cities to the incidence of disease and to the worsening quality of life of the inhabitants, while painfully slow, were both curative and preventive in nature. Medically speaking, the city's abundance of potential patients and the wide variety of diseases they were afflicted with consistently attracted large concentrations of medical practitioners and specialists. Likewise, a large proportion of the country's new professional medical institutions, the medical schools and societies, were founded in urban areas. In effect, the city became the focal point of young America's attempts to catch up with European formal medicine. By the Civil War, several of the country's municipalities—particularly Philadelphia, Boston, New York, and Charleston—were already considered by some to have gone a considerable distance toward accomplishing this objective.

The expansion of medical care facilities was a large part of the cities' efforts. Almshouses, for their part, multiplied considerably after the Revolution. Typically these were grim institutions. J. H. Miller, physician to the Baltimore Almshouse, in 1835 referred to such places as "humanity's commons, where the useless and incurable are turned out to die." Never adequate substitutes for hospitals, their bare wards afforded few comforts and few cures. However, given the variety of ailments among the inmates, they did provide clinical experience for many a city physician and medical student.

Scattered new general hospitals also began to appear during the post-Revolutionary and antebellum periods. Unlike the almshouses, such institutions tended not to admit incurables, but they were open to paying patients as well as "respectable" charity patients. However, only after the Civil War did they become numerous enough to be considered typical parts of America's urban medical habitat. One of the reasons for this delay was the relative lack of interest on the part of the upper and middle classes, most of whom continued to have physicians treat them at their homes. By contrast, the poor, especially among the new immigrants, took full advantage of the existing institutions. In late antebellum New Orleans, for instance, less than 2 percent of the patients at Charity Hospital were found to be natives of Louisiana; most of the rest were recent immigrants.

Along with the general hospitals, cities also began to accumulate a variety of other medical care institutions during the nineteenth century. Among these were scattered small hospitals for blacks and free dispensaries for the poor. Private infirmaries or clinics arose to deal with eye and ear diseases, obstetrics, lung ailments, and other conditions. Asylums for the blind and for "deaf and dumb" persons began to spring up soon after the War of 1812. Asylums or hospitals for the mentally ill also multiplied from that time. Generally located in or near the cities, the latter institutions increasingly utilized the new "moral treatment," a therapy that emphasized humane methods, together with the maintenance of a pleasant and uplifting environment. The early peak of this asylum-building movement came during the late 1840s with the remarkable crusade of the New Englander, Dorothea Lynde Dix, to create more such institutions throughout the Union.

If the leaders of most cities were slow in building medical care institutions, they were even more dilatory in providing public health facilities or services. However, they normally continued the various general sanitary ordinances, though these were typically ineffective and sporadic in nature as well as inadequate to the demands of rapidly expanding communities. Larger cities also began to offer free public vaccination early in the nineteenth century, and a few made it compulsory later in the century. Publication of periodic bills of mortality, prepared from undertakers' or sextons' reports and arranged by causes of death, was resumed after the Revolution and spread to other cities, though they did not begin to be systematically prepared or scientifically utilized for public health work until almost mid-century.

While some cities and towns nominally had standing boards of health, the more usual practice for many years was simply to appoint such boards to handle specific epidemics and then allow them to go out of existence. Most large cities occasionally utilized medical society committees to look into particular health problems. And ultimately they took on nuisance inspectors and quarantine officials as city employees, often part time and not necessarily controlled by the boards of health. But such positions were highly vulnerable to politics. Public health reformers, among them New York's John Griscom, a physician, and Boston's Lemuel Shattuck, a merchant, in the 1840s began urging the creation of permanent health boards and departments with full-time trained professionals in active charge. This proved to be an elusive ideal; prior to the Civil War, Providence was almost the only city to have made such arrangements.

Largely outside the purview of the health boards, but of major significance for urban health, were the cities' arrangements for obtaining water and for the disposal of large-scale human, animal, and industrial wastes. Such provisions were notoriously too little and too late throughout this period. Nevertheless, civic leaders began to realize that, while small towns could continue to leave such arrangements to individual property owners, large modern cities required well-coordinated public provisions. Moreover, a considerable segment of the late-eighteenth- and early-nineteenth-century medical community agreed that there was probably a close correlation between filthy environments and certain crowd diseases. While this theory continued to lack proof, city officials and reformers in America, as in Great Britain and Europe, were strongly guided by it in their arguments for improved urban sanitary arrangements. The antebellum needs were such, in fact, as to lead America's larger cities gradually to commit themselves to the launching of what ultimately became huge, complex, and enormously costly sanitary works.

Individual wells continued to furnish water for some city families throughout most of the nineteenth century. But service from private water companies—either by wagon or from reservoirs through pipes—rapidly expanded after the Revolution. Since these supplies in turn were seldom adequate or reliable, certain cities were eventually forced to construct their own water systems. Benjamin Latrobe designed a successful waterworks for Philadelphia in 1799. And, during the 1840s, great reservoir and aqueduct systems were built in New York and Boston and inaugurated with much pomp. However, relatively few other municipal systems were added before the Civil War.

As soon as abundant water supplies became available, more effective drain systems also proved increasingly feasible. By the 1840s, Boston, Philadelphia, New York, and a few other cities had begun construction of underground sewer systems in downtown areas. As they did so, householders were encouraged to connect their house drains to them and to install indoor plumbing. However, this remained unfeasible for most city dwellings for some time, while landlords often strenuously resisted the step. As a result, the malodorous outdoor privy continued as a conspicuous and offensive feature of urban life for the rest of the nineteenth century and into the twentieth. And, as long as the privies remained, provisions had to be made for the regular removal of the night soil, measures that generally left much to be desired.

Ever larger enterprises also came into being to try to keep city streets clean and to dispose of the growing quantities of garbage and rubbish. In many instances, such wastes were simply hauled by contractors to the closest rivers or lakes. Other cities utilized dumps on the outskirts or, in the case of garbage, pig farms. All such measures had serious drawbacks: the collections of wastes tended to be irregular; the vehicles used were generally unhygienic in the extreme; while the dumps or other deposit sites became chronically malodorous and unaesthetic sources of air and water pollution.

American city officials by and large faced these basic sanitary problems with much reluctance. By the 1860s, however, some had begun to arrange for legislative authority and financing for the large projects. They had started to bring in the varied engineers, contractors, and builders that were required for such work. And they were looking increasingly to the physicians for justification.

As in Great Britain a generation or so earlier, it was evident that these mid-nineteenth-century American sanitary stirrings and energies did not come from city officials and a few medical men alone. Clergymen, businessmen, statisticians, members of do-good societies, and others were also interested and involved. By the 1850s, representatives of many of these groups had started to come together in local sanitary groups. And at the end of that decade a series of national quarantine and sanitary conventions demonstrated that this early American sanitary movement was gaining in force and unity.

The Commercial Factor in Medicine and Health

However much the city's medical development and health environment were shaped by professional impulses and reform initiatives, they were also strongly influenced by the nineteenth century's intense preoccupation with business, industry, and economic matters. In fact, formal medical activity in each of the habitats reflected America's prevailing commercialism in various ways. The relationships were sometimes ambivalent. For instance, the rise of a well-to-do urban middle class had much to do with stimulating the increase in numbers of physicians as well as with filling the spas and water-cure establishments with customers. At the same time, the slow build-up of hospitals, sewers, and water works related closely to the gradual improvement in the cities' economic capacity.

As in other countries, American cities vying with each other for commercial and economic preeminence often extended their competition to health matters. Since trade was easily discouraged by the presence of communicable disease, business interests tended to try to suppress news about epidemics of smallpox, yellow fever, or cholera in their respective communities, and to resist the imposition of quarantines. This tendency to deny the presence of disease eventually became part of a booster syndrome in which a city's positive health attractions and medical institutions were not only publicized but habitually exaggerated as part of the competition with other cities. As the nineteenth century went on, such boosterism was often made more difficult by the unattractive practices of certain businesses—by the refusal of city landlords to improve their unsanitary tenements, for instance, or by the increasingly flagrant pollution of watercourses by factories. Other members of the business community, however, out of self-interest or recognizing the negative effect that such practices had on the city's image and commerce, often became active supporters of improved water supply facilities, public sewer systems, and other public health measures.

For the individual nineteenth-century physician, the pursuit of a medical practice also had its economic aspects. As a small businessperson he had to cope with office records and with the collection of accounts, though he did not do very well at either. He frequently found himself in competition for patients with one or more sectarian practitioners, and sometimes made less money than they did. Although some city doctors amassed considerable wealth, the average practitioner throughout the century was far from well-off. Many continued to supplement their income by selling or endorsing medications, farming, running stores, or speculating in real estate.

Medical institutions likewise frequently had roles as business entities. Some small private hospitals were run for profit. And proprietary medical schools also were run frankly as profit-making bodies. While there was a high rate of failure among the latter, new schools quickly took their places, launched in many cases with extravagant promotional literature. Medical journals, in turn, which were frequently founded by members of the proprietary faculties, proved even more ephemeral than the schools as business enterprises; many of them failed after only one or two issues. However, the total numbers continued to increase.

Native medical book publishing was generally more successful, economically. This business expanded dramatically after the Revolution, largely in direct response to the multiplication of physicians. During the first half of the nineteenth century, the reprinting of British medical works formed a considerable proportion of this business. American medical leaders repeatedly nagged their colleagues about the dearth and low quality of the books by native medical authors. But improvement remained slow throughout the antebellum period.

The emergence of domestic life insurance during the 1840s brought into being another large-scale and commercially profitable enterprise that had important medical ramifications. With it, some physicians gained added income as insurance inspectors. Applicants for policies, meanwhile, were made more conscious of their physical condition by the need to pass a medical examination. And health departments began to receive both monetary and statistical support from the insurance companies for their preventive activities.

The antebellum medical scene was also increasingly shaped by industrial developments. A number of native industries emerged as producers of health-related goods, first on a small scale but eventually growing in size. Through the early post-Revolutionary decades, most of America's needs for drugs, as well as for various items of medical equipment, continued to be filled by imports. In the case of drugs, individual apothecaries did a limited amount of compounding. From the 1820s and 1830s onward, however, small native laboratories, many of them in Philadelphia, began producing a variety of chemicals, patent medicines, and other preparations. Similarly, in small shops, American artisans designed and began the production of a growing range of surgical, dental, and other instruments and equipment. A consistent demand for these different products ensured the success of many of these shops and the conspicuous growth of some, particularly during and after the Civil War.

Throughout the century, medicine benefited from the invention and development of rapid modes of transportation. The railway facilitated patient travel to resorts or spas. It enabled itinerant healers, bonesetters, and patent-medicine salesmen to cover more territory, and it permitted peripatetic physicians to teach in medical schools hundreds of miles apart in successive terms. Rapid transportation and, from the 1840s, rapid communication in the form of the telegraph, also aided in the diffusion of new medical ideas, while the development of efficient mail and express systems revolutionized the distribution of drugs, medical books and journals, and instruments.

In part because of the relatively late development of industrialism in the United States, Americans were slow in manifesting concern for its various adverse health consequences, potential or real. However, after 1830 numerous instances of the deleterious effects of industrialism began to come to public attention. Reports of train wrecks and exploding steamships multiplied. News of the mangling or loss of limbs in these accidents and in factory machinery became commonplace. Reformers claimed that long hours of work, poor ventilation, and lack of exercise in the mills of Lowell and other early factory towns so impaired the health of respectable female workers that many left their jobs and returned to the farms to die prematurely. At the same time, other observers noted that workers' housing in mill communities was frequently deficient, while the industrial pollution of soil, air, and water supplies was rapidly worsening.

Throughout the period, most members of the upper classes tended to be insensitive to the hazards of the unhealthiest and most dangerous industrial jobs, such as those of miners, railway gangs, or construction workers. Reflecting this, state and federal government intervention or regulation to improve health or safety conditions was rarely considered. At best it remained something that most people wanted to put off as long as possible.

Medicine, Health, and the Reluctant State

Only rarely did state or federal governments act on any kind of health-related concerns, particularly in the early post-Revolutionary decades. Even city governments became involved only reluctantly in such matters. Wherever possible, the latter tended to turn over such concerns—quarantine inspection or public vaccination, for example—to local medical society committees or individual physicians. Nevertheless, as their populations and problems multiplied, cities had no choice but to gradually accumulate both health responsibilities and medical bureaucracies. By the time of the 1849 cholera outbreak, Philadelphia's Board of Health by itself was said to have taken on enough employees "to conduct the affairs of the South American Republics."

By contrast, state governments up to that time had scarcely begun to acquire staffs for health-related purposes. One level removed as they were from local crises or problems of most kinds, the states, despite their inherent powers, were uniformly slow in assuming operational roles in medicine or public health. It was not necessarily the result of a prevailing laissez-faire philosophy, for commercial interests did manage to obtain allocations of public funds. However, legislatures were understandably reluctant to legislate on medical matters as long as medicine failed to speak with a single authoritative voice. And they had no incentive to consider public health programs until their territories included sizeable urban areas with serious sanitary problems.

The states' initial hesitations over the licensing of medical practitioners can be understood in the light of the virtually total absence of medical oversight by the British during the colonial period. The solution adopted by most early-nineteenth-century legislatures in this matter was not to create state agencies for the purpose but to delegate the licensing authority to private bodies, i.e., to the existing state and local medical societies. At the time, these were all orthodox in their medical orientation. However, beginning in the 1830s, sectarian interests became strong enough to challenge and ultimately force the repeal of most of these state arrangements. Ultimately, after the Civil War, new pressures to resume state licensing built up. But by then the prevalent opinion favored direct licensure by state boards of one sort or another, and with the boards empowered to examine sectarian as well as orthodox applicants.

During the antebellum period, most state governments became involved in medical care to some extent, chiefly the operation of public asylums or hospitals for the blind, deaf, and mentally ill. Other instances included the engaging of physicians to handle sickness among prison inmates. Moreover, New York, Louisiana, and other states, as part of their quarantine provisions, engaged physicians to inspect immigrants, hospitalize those who were ill, and manage other activities.

Nevertheless, public health reformers of the period generally considered the states to be backward in their commitments to health. In 1845, Edward Jarvis of Massachusetts summed up the argument: "Our governments . . . have legislated for property, but not for life. They have cared for the lands, the cattle, the money of their constituents, but not for their health and longevity." As steps toward redressing the balance, several states began to limit the length of the working day for child laborers. Moreover, following the lead of Massachusetts, a dozen states, mostly in the East, around 1850 launched new attempts to register births and deaths, though few such systems worked at all well until the twentieth century. Similarly, Lemuel Shattuck in 1850 provided the blueprint for a comprehensive state board of health for Massachusetts, but it proved premature, as did Louisiana's slightly later attempt to create such a body.

The federal government's early role in medical matters, like that of the states, was tentative and spotty. Actually, given the lack of a specific medical mandate in the Constitution, the health-related activities that were undertaken in the century after the Revolution were little more than incidental parts of other kinds of governmental functions. However, several of these activities, though expanding only slowly in size, took on progressively greater medical significance.

The armed forces, of course, had to assemble and administer large temporary medical establishments while prosecuting four major wars between 1775 and 1865. But these were rapidly done away with at the end of hostilities, leaving only small peacetime cadres and facilities. The Army created a central medical department for its permanent forces in 1818, while the Navy did so in 1842. The former coordinated the assignment of medical officers to troop detachments operating along and beyond the frontier and supervised hospitals and medical personnel of the tiny garrisons. The Navy, in turn, provided medical personnel for its larger warships and, after the War of 1812, began erecting permanent hospitals at various port cities.

In both military services, medical officers often had leisure to collect natural history or anthropological specimens. And a few, prominent among them William Beaumont, made original medical observations of importance. The collected medical and meteorological reports of the Army's antebellum medical officers, moreover, provided particularly significant information on the presumed relationships of weather and disease.

Apart from military needs, the federal government in 1798 also accepted responsibility for the medical care of the nation's merchant seamen. With funds collected from shipmasters, the Treasury Department originally provided temporary or contract facilities for sick or disabled sailors in the principal American ports. By the War of 1812, however, it was beginning to purchase or build its own marine hospitals. After the mid-1830s the Department also located such institutions in the Mississippi Valley area to provide care for riverboat men and Great Lakes sailors. Designed in the period's eclectic architectural styles, the marine hospitals included some of the nation's largest and most imposing antebellum medical care edifices. But no central medical bureau to coordinate them existed until after the Civil War.

A federal contribution to the study of disease in the United States was made possible by successive enlargements in the scope of the decennial censuses. The first four censuses, from 1790 through 1820, did not include any health-related inquiries. However, several such inquiries were subsequently added: in 1830 to determine the numbers of the deaf, "dumb," and blind; in 1840 to enumerate the insane and idiots; and in 1850 to obtain mortality figures. The full social and scientific potential of these inquiries was not realized for a good many years, due principally to deficiencies in the enumeration processes. Nevertheless, almost from the beginning some of the data collected

were utilized in effective and sometimes inflammatory ways to enhance regional medical and political positions in late antebellum
America.

At every stage of the early national experience, many Americans
assumed that there were differences in salubrity from one region to
another. Transplanted physicians maintained that the new sections
of the country varied from the older regions they had come from,
both in the nature of their diseases and in the special medicines
appropriate in treating them. Some Revolutionary Era Americans
stressed the dissimilarities of their diseases from those of England;
midwesterners and southerners subsequently saw differences in their
regions both from the East and from Europe. Trans-Appalachian residents during the 1830s and 1840s seemed to talk as much about their
gargantuan diseases as about their outsized folk heroes, Mike Fink
and Davy Crockett. And certain western physicians of that period
claimed that only they understood how to utilize outsized heroic
therapies in dealing with such diseases. They considered eastern textbooks and medical schools to be useless in preparing doctors for
practice in the West.

This viewpoint did not prevail universally either in the Mississippi
valley or further west. But it found a highly congenial soil in the
South during the final two antebellum decades. There the concept of
a distinctive southern medicine was employed to gain support for
the recently founded medical schools and medical journals of the
region. But some southern physicians went on to link the growth of
these institutions, particularly the medical schools, with the region's
solidifying political position and its views on slavery. As such, the
proponents of the so-called "states-rights medicine," fire-eaters such
as Samuel Cartwright, went to increasing lengths to undermine the
reputations of the popular northern medical schools in the eyes of
southern medical students. It was a tactic that culminated in 1859
with a substantial exodus of such students from Philadelphia and
New York schools.

The Civil War proved to be by far the country's largest and most
devastating medical event of the nineteenth century. As such it led
to an unprecedented involvement in medical matters by government.
Over the four bloody years of the War, the Union and Confederate
governments coped with similar health problems and built up parallel
military medical establishments to handle them. To supplement their
tiny nuclei of regular-army medical officers, they brought together
large numbers of volunteer doctors, pharmacists, and other personnel. They organized ambulance corps, assembled hospital trains, and
built vast general hospitals. They made at least nominal medical in-
spections of recruits. Both sides were constantly trying to obtain med-

ical supplies, the Confederacy the more urgently because of the Union's blockade. Leaders of both worried about camp sanitation; despite their best efforts to heed the lessons of Crimea, the deaths from diseases mounted above those from battle wounds. And, as England's Florence Nightingale had done in the Crimean War, civilians on both sides organized important medical relief organizations to furnish volunteer nurses and otherwise aid the troops.

The combined mortality toll of the two sides during the Civil War amounted to something over 600,000, while additional thousands died later of wounds, injuries, and diseases. Moreover, the overall devastation caused by the war, particularly in the South, further affected peoples' health and well-being in large portions of the country for years to come. Institutionally, the wartime closure or destruction of southern medical schools, journals, and other institutions set back the region's production of physicians and its capacity to care for its citizens. Some southern doctors moved to the North after the war in order to regain their livelihoods. Among the southern whites as a whole, many were so impoverished as to become seriously weakened by malnutrition and immobilized by such endemic conditions as malaria and hookworm disease.

The blacks were even worse off. Despite reconstruction relief efforts, large numbers of the freed slaves were left homeless, jobless, hungry, poorly clothed, and highly vulnerable to disease. The wartime Freedmen's Inquiry Commission had wondered what the chances were "of Negro survival in a white-dominated society." And the extremely high subsequent rates of black morbidity and mortality gave continuing pertinence to that question throughout the rest of the century and beyond.

The war likewise had deep-seated effects throughout the country on certain branches of medicine. Many volunteer medical officers on leaving the service went back to their communities with a greatly enhanced competence in surgery; others with a new appreciation for hygiene and sanitation. Such specialties as pathology and neurology were equally advanced. Pharmaceutical manufacturing, despite Surgeon-General Hammond's attempt to limit the northern army's use of calomel, emerged from the war as a big business. The war's immense toll of amputations provided considerable stimulus to the refinement and manufacture of prosthetics in the United States. Similarly, the knowledge of hospital management that was gained during the war greatly facilitated the postwar organization of new civilian hospitals. And the employment of female nurses in wartime hospitals helped show the way to their increased utilization in civil institutions.

Another major consequence of the Civil War was to leave the

Federal government with a permanently expanded role in medical matters. The United States Soldiers Home was created to care for disabled veterans, with branches ultimately in various states. The new Freedmen's Bureau provided a certain amount of medical care to blacks, while the Bureau of Indian Affairs continued to do so for Indians on reservations. The wartime Morrill Act, meanwhile, with land grants to the states, stimulated the rise of state universities around the country, and with them the creation of agricultural research stations and the further multiplication of medical schools, veterinary schools, and science departments.

Although the wartime medical apparatus of both the Union and Confederate forces was largely dismantled, the Surgeon-General's office of the Northern Army emerged from hostilities with a number of continuing projects which took on considerable significance for postwar America's medical community. The office's wartime collection of pathological specimens and other objects was quickly arranged and put on display in a permanent medical museum, an institution that took on significant research and teaching functions. Meanwhile, in a project that took nearly a quarter-century to complete, Joseph J. Woodward, George Otis, and other medical officers gradually processed the vast accumulation of wartime medical records for a massive published account of the war's medical and surgical history. During the same period, John Shaw Billings built up the Surgeon-General's Library almost from scratch into the country's largest medical library.

These and related activities were housed until the late 1880s in Washington, D.C., in what had been Ford's Theatre, the building where President Lincoln was assassinated. In this structure, Woodward, Billings, and their colleagues also carried on significant research in pathology, microscopy, hospital design and ventilation, vital statistics, and other areas of medicine. The researches of these government physicians, together with their management of the increasingly useful library and museum facilities, combined to turn Ford's Theatre into America's most influential single center of medical activity during the immediate post–Civil War years. Moreover, the successive volumes of the *Medical and Surgical History* gained no little admiration in European as well as American medical circles. However, some of the findings of mid-nineteenth-century Europe's brilliant scientific community began to suggest that there were certain limitations in that publication. They also pointed up remaining gaps in America's medical and scientific capabilities.

CHAPTER 3

THE ASCENDANT NATION:
TRANSFORMATIONS IN MEDICINE
AND HEALTH, 1865–1940

THE ENDING of the Civil War enabled the United States to come back together as a power that had to be reckoned with, militarily and politically. In population it was already one of the largest nations in the Western world. The enormous productivity of its agriculture and industry had made it one of the wealthiest. But there was agreement that some aspects of national life—among them, higher education, science, and medicine—still required considerable development before the country could be said to have shed the persistent onus of deficiency that had accompanied the early underdeveloped status.

In 1865 the country's civilian medical life was still relatively simple, though growing in scale. Medical practice continued to be divided among mainline and sectarian groups, all of them still largely ineffective in both their organizations and their therapies and hostile toward each other. Medicine was far more devoted to the art of health care than to the search for knowledge, and it centered in the individual practitioner rather than in institutions or governments. Still, in almost every respect, it had been slowly changing. In fact, once the destructive war came to an end, the forces of change became so potent as to transform almost every aspect of medicine quickly and radically, sometimes virtually beyond recognition.

Health and Medicine in Changing Habitats

The political, economic, social, and industrial energies unleashed in post–Civil War America were particularly powerful. Acting together, they rapidly altered the familiar environments of health and disease of a large majority of the people and at the same time profoundly affected the circumstances of medical practice and health care. Demographic forces were formidable by themselves. The still substantial birthrate, together, until the 1920s, with an enormously expanding immigration from abroad, ensured a level of population increase that underlay many of the other changes. Population increase, moreover, made for the emergence of a reservoir of disease that was unprecedented in scale in the nation. At the same time, the constant movement of people into towns and cities was already changing the American population from a people that was predominantly rural in character to one that was increasingly urban in composition. In the West, the incoming of additional white settlers accelerated the formation of new states, hastened the end of effective Indian resistance, and in 1890 brought about official acknowledgment of the end of the country's frontier.

In every section of the country, in the period after 1865, Americans accelerated the processes that were modifying their habitats and health environments. On the creative side, they sped up the formation and development of the basic legal and governmental structures, social and cultural institutions, and educational systems that underlie and help support medicine. At the same time, Americans expanded their often rapacious exploitation of the land, forests, and other natural resources. And, with the financial tycoons and "robber barons" of the Gilded Age, many broadened their search for wealth, pushed for ever more intensive industrialization, and generally promoted the accumulation of people in urban settings. Still, for all the changes, America remained a nation with a number of distinctive kinds of habitats.

One of these continued to be the transient environment that was home or workplace for very large numbers of people. These still included numerous migrants and immigrants looking for places to settle. They also included professional travelers—somewhat fewer western explorers, soldiers, hunters, and itinerants than previously, perhaps, but more traveling salesmen and railroad conductors. New homeless men as well as hoboes multiplied after every economic disruption, while certain distinct social groups were at times impelled by chronic hardship or natural disaster to move en masse in the attempt to improve their lot. Among such dislocations was the large-scale movement of southern blacks to northern cities that began around 1915 and the trek of the "Okies" from the dust bowl of the central plains to California in the 1930s.

While some of the circumstances of the transient life changed after 1865, they did not usually make for better health. To be sure, ongoing improvements in transportation greatly reduced the time needed for individuals to move from one place to another. Moreover, the continued mushrooming of new towns, particularly in the West, theoretically made medical attention more available to transients or travelers. Nevertheless, the quality of life remained low for many such individuals, with greater than average vulnerability to disease, irregular access to medical services, and little money or credit to pay for any such services beyond those provided by charities.

The farm, under changing conditions, continued to provide a more mixed health environment. This was partly due to the farmers' perennial vulnerability to the vagaries of nature as well as to the increasing effects of market fluctuations and governmental policies. Drought and debt led to poor health along the "Middle Border" of the Dakotas as surely as comparable circumstances did in the South or New England. For the more fortunate, the increasing use of mechanical planters, reapers, threshing-machines, and eventually tractors greatly reduced the backbreaking labors of farm life while immensely enlarging the commercial productivity of farms. But the multiplication of machines also greatly increased the risk of serious accidents.

For most of this period, however, horses, mules, and oxen continued to play far larger labor roles on the American farm than tractors, while on many farms the maintenance or production of animals for the food market became an ever larger enterprise. Given the immense numbers of such animals, together with the additional large numbers used in other habitats for transportation or kept as pets, the effective medical care of animals became a matter of increasing economic urgency. During the post–Civil War period, with the creation of state landgrant colleges and the emergence of proprietary veterinary medical schools, the early era of self-trained farriers and blacksmiths utilizing popular veterinary handbooks steadily gave way to one of better qualified practitioners. The specialty was rapidly organized along professional lines with the creation of specialized veterinary journals and professional societies. And by 1900 veterinary practice had begun to be transformed in character and effectiveness by the spread of modern laboratory science. Within a few decades, veterinary scientists found the means of controlling hog cholera, Texas cattle fever, trichinosis, tuberculosis, and several other destructive diseases affecting animals and sometimes people as well. This helped bring about, in the twentieth century, a marked upgrading of the public image of the veterinary practitioner.

Some contributions of late-nineteenth- and early-twentieth-century technology, such as electricity and indoor plumbing, came to rural America too late to benefit the lives or health of many farmers during this period. But the telephone, improved roads, and automobiles did begin to reduce the farmer's painful sense of isolation and to make the medical resources of nearby towns or cities more rapidly accessible. In addition, such organizations as the Grange and the Farm Bureau did much to improve the quality of farm life by organizing recreational activities, promoting better hygienic practices, publicizing new modes of preserving foods, and advocating better diets.

The health environment of the small town was even more immediately affected by the burgeoning industrialism and technology. Villagers acquired a variety of their own machines, along with the attendant accident hazards, as they established small shops and industries. The coming of electricity brought streetlights as well as radios, telephones, and other household appliances. The quality of life and health in post–Civil War houses and public buildings, meanwhile, also benefited from improvements in heating, ventilation, and plumbing.

Formal medical services in the small town continued to center mainly upon the individual general practitioners. However, in time, hospitals, clinics, or sanatoria began to appear in the more populous places. Also, depending on size, the villages were increasingly likely to have their own druggists, dentists, practical nurses, and veterinary doctors. Ultimately, many of the physicians served also as local health officers. At the same time, under guidelines of state departments of health, towns began providing garbage collection services as well as installing their own water and sewerage systems. As these were completed, the historic but unhygienic privy vaults slowly gave way, in many areas, to modern indoor facilities.

Even more than the farmers, residents of small towns found that their medical options were broadened by the innovations in transportation. The coming of train or trolley service as well as the improvement of highways greatly facilitated the access of townspeople to medical specialists and hospitals in nearby cities. Eventually, such facilities opened up opportunities for recreational travel, both to the city and the country. In the small towns, physicians were often among the earliest to purchase automobiles. Difficulties in reaching their rural patients in the new conveyances subsequently turned some of them into strong agitators for the improvement of roads. One such doctor, William L. Higgins, in the 1920s successfully ran for state senator under the motto, "Get Connecticut Out of the Mud."

Contrasting sharply with the prototypical, rather sleepy rural villages were those small towns that were substantially taken over by aggressive industries or that were specifically organized as company towns or camps. These ranged from occasional well-planned and more or less paternalistic communities such as Lowell or Pullman to those that were hastily thrown together and harshly run in the pursuit of profit. Numerically, such towns and their sprawling industries increased greatly after the Civil War, and a low level of health environment prevailed in most of them. All too often, the streets of the towns were lined with workers' houses that were packed together, dingy, in poor repair, lacking in modern plumbing, and looking out on mounting piles of industrial wastes. The atmosphere was typically smoky, the sanitary and public health provisions inadequate, and the recreation facilities few. The principal employment of the inhabitants, moreover, tended to be in the most dangerous and unhealthful occupations of the new industrial age. For adults, these included not only the endlessly repetitive operations in certain factories but hazardous and backbreaking tasks in mines, forests, quarries, meat-packing firms, iron works, and flour mills, as well as pressure-filled jobs on speeded-up assembly lines. However, as late as 1900, some two million American children under fifteen were also working for a living, a circumstance that bore directly on the painful disease and mortality rates of their age group.

Correction of the worst evils of the industrial environments came slowly. The lethal health effects of certain processes and toxic waste deposits, in fact, received little attention from society or government until the mid-twentieth century. Safety provisions in factories, however, did improve to some extent between the 1870s and World War II, under the stimulus of public health programs, workers' compensation laws, and other social legislation. Particularly important after 1900 in drawing attention to the numerous medical and other hazards in the workplace were the surveys and researches carried out by Edith Hamilton and a small number of other state and federal investigators.

At the same time, some medical care facilities and services began to appear in the company towns, though those provided by the companies themselves were often regarded by workers as attempts to undercut the labor unions. While mid-nineteenth-century industries generally called in physicians from nearby communities to treat injured workers, following the Civil War larger firms—particularly railroads, mining companies, and steel manufacturers—increasingly retained their own physicians. By around 1900 such firms, especially those in isolated areas, provided varied but usually minimal medical services, sometimes through contract arrangements and sometimes including dependents of workers as well. A few of them, notably the railroads, began operating their own hospitals and clinics, as did some unions, especially in the West. Industries also began, in the early 1900s, as part of scientific management, to experiment with preventive occupational hygiene, a movement that expanded in several directions in the decades before World War II.

The health environment of cities was even more profoundly altered than that of the small town by the rapid spread of industrialism. Here the impact of the multiplying factories and of the new products of technology was intensified by the coincidental continuing inrush of huge additional populations. To be sure, in a few places early-twentieth-century environmentalists and planners sought ways to keep peoples' living environments healthfully distant from the factories and their associated evils. In far more instances, at least where the poor and laboring classes were concerned, the residential areas and industries tended to rise in close proximity. However, even the upper social classes were by no means wholly insulated from the effects of rapid urbanization and industrialization. In fact, the neurologist George M. Beard attributed the vague "nervous" complaints that were widespread around the turn of the century, particularly among women of these classes, directly to stresses brought on by these environments.

The expansion of urban businesses and industries furnished employment for many of the new inhabitants. However, this advantage was substantially offset in cities by a constant compression in the amount of peoples' living space, by a continuing hygienic deterioration in the older housing, and by chronic shortages of public parks. Large numbers of city dwellers, in any case, were always unemployed, poverty-stricken, and vulnerable to illness. The tenement districts where many lived continued to be known as the areas with the worst hygienic conditions as well as some of the nation's highest infant mortality rates. Meanwhile, large numbers of urban workers lost their health working at certain low-paying jobs, notoriously in sweatshops or the "dusty trades"—milling, stone-cutting, wood-turning, and others.

The better of the new public buildings, factories, and residences that sprang up in late-nineteenth- and early-twentieth-century cities tended to be increasingly well heated as well as better furnished with running water and plumbing. However, the quality of living of almost all classes of citizens continued to be adversely affected by the coal smoke that dirtied peoples' homes and choked their lungs, at least up to the advent of oil-burning and electrical furnaces. The replacement of horses by automobiles, trucks, and buses was an enormous contribution to clean streets as well as to the reduction of flies. However, the new vehicles also filled the urban air with increasingly dangerous concentrations of toxic fumes. The coming of electric streetcars, subways, and railways, in turn, facilitated the travel of many tenement dwellers to their factory jobs; but they also made it increasingly feasible for the growing middle and upper classes to avoid much of the city's hygienic drawbacks by living in spacious and salubrious homes in the suburbs.

The various disparities between the well-to-do and the poor of the post–Civil War cities carried over to the formal health-related resources that each segment of the population had at its disposal. During this period, sanitary services continued to spread throughout the cities, but the well-to-do sections were generally connected to sewer and water lines before the tenement areas were. Cities continued to attract large numbers of every conceivable variety of medical practitioner and health professional. But most of the traditional healers, midwives, and folk practitioners tended to concentrate in the less affluent sections, while specialists and other highly educated physicians gravitated to the wealthy. The differences in quality of the health-related attention received by the various classes were all too apparent and were increasingly well documented, as in New York City by the muckraking journalist Jacob Riis. Moreover, in the attempt to reduce those differences to some small degree, slum dwellers were made the targets of health service programs initiated by numerous well-meaning organizations—settlement houses, visiting nurse groups, schools, and other private and public agencies—as well as by governments.

Among the most sweeping of the post–Civil War changes in formal health care arrangements was the coming of age of hospital care and services. This phenomenon amounted, in fact, to a revolution that affected all populations in the urban habitat, and to a lesser degree those in the various other habitats as well. Following the Civil War the numbers of such institutions proliferated from hardly more than 100 hospitals in all parts of the nation in 1870, not including mental asylums, to over 6,000 in the next fifty years, largely in cities. Most of them were general hospitals, but there were also various special institutions.

The burst of hospital construction owed a good deal to the era's demographic events and pressures. In 1876, when Philadelphia's Centennial Exhibition opened, institutions in many communities were still caring for large numbers of Civil War wounded. It was thus still timely for the Army Medical Department to set up a display at the Exhibition which featured models of Civil War hospitals and equipment. The Department also exhibited the far-smaller hospitals that it was by then using in the military's tiny peacetime posts, mostly in the West. But in 1876 the Indian wars were nearly over. And in any case, it had become evident that there were now far greater needs for civilian than for military hospitals, and most conspicuously in the cities.

Among the post–Civil War responses to these needs was the acceleration of moves to transform almshouses into hospitals for the needy as well as to erect new city hospitals. Far more extensive, however, was the expansion of philanthropic institutions, of hospitals that were typically sponsored, financed, and managed by churches and other humanitarian groups. Elite doctors were often active in pushing for and organizing such institutions, and they subsequently gained much influence in them over the years. At the same time, other hospitals sprang up that were entirely organized and run by groups of physicians. As in earlier decades, some of the new hospitals were built or controlled by homeopaths and other sects, though after World War I most of these affiliated with the regulars. Whatever their affiliation or nature, the hospitals became increasingly prominent physical features of the health environment of late-nineteenth- and twentieth-century American cities. While all too many were drab and functional in appearance, at least some had architectural distinction, and in time a good many deliberately reflected the opulence of the period in decor, furnishings, and services.

For most of the nineteenth century and even beyond, the public dispensaries also remained numerous in many cities, where they made more significant contributions than most hospitals in caring for the sick poor. However, as general hospitals became more numerous and came to include outpatient facilities, the dispensaries began to disappear. At the same time, specialty clinics of all kinds increased greatly in number and often in size. Some institutions, such as those developed by the Mayo and Menninger families, eventually gained considerable reputations and attracted far-flung clienteles.

Mental hospitals also continued to multiply. Under the steady crush of large numbers of patients, many humane elements of the old "moral" treatment had to be all but abandoned by the late-nineteenth century, as most institutions reverted to essentially custodial roles. Some new therapies were introduced as they became available. The use of psychotherapy and psychoanalysis, in particular, began to spread soon after 1900, and other measures later on. But all too often the institutions were dismal, even forbidding, components of the urban environment, establishments that offered few rays of hope to patients or their families.

One type of special hospital that emerged during this period did seem to offer some hope, its sponsors thought, if only by taking patients out of their insalubrious urban environments. This was the tuberculosis sanatorium, with its heavy emphasis on fresh air, rest, and abundant food, but eventually also with such surgical procedures as artificial pneumothorax, or lung collapse. The American prototype of this institution was established by Edward Trudeau in 1884 at Saranac Lake, in New York's Adirondack Mountains. Trudeau's sanatorium was followed, over the next half-century or so, by similar establishments in other mountainous areas around the country. Some of these were organized and run by health departments, churches, or voluntary health organizations. But the largest number were private money-making ventures.

Generally speaking, the hospitals of the late-nineteenth century were better managed than their predecessors. Their officers increasingly organized themselves into specialty organizations and established professional journals. Most significant, their patients tended to get steadily improved care.

Of central importance in bringing this about was the reform of nursing, a step originally stimulated largely by upper-class women who had come under the influence of England's "lady with a lamp," Florence Nightingale. Among other results, their agitation helped lead to the establishment of urgently needed nurses' training schools. The earliest of these were formed at New York's Bellevue Hospital and a few other hospitals in the early 1870s; by 1900 over 400 such institutions had been created. At the same time further steps to upgrade nursing were being taken, including the formation of professional societies, the creation of journals, and, in nearly every state, the establishment of nurse examiners.

A further signal improvement in the late-nineteenth-century hospital, one that grew at least partly from the Nightingale precepts, was a new insistence on cleanliness in the wards, which occurred at about the same time as the successive introduction of antiseptic and aseptic practices into the operating rooms. The British surgeon Joseph Lister came to America during the nation's centennial year with much acclaim to talk about his antiseptic procedures. But it was nearly another decade before surgeons in large numbers adopted them in the United States.

During these same decades, the refinement of anesthesia in surgery, by further reducing the patient's burden of pain, drastically improved the hospital's internal atmosphere and made operations of all kinds infinitely more supportable, both to patients and surgeons. As time went on, noticeable improvements were made also in such matters as hospital diet, lighting, ventilation, and supplies of medication and instruments, as well as in the provision of luxury services for patients who could pay for them. The introduction of the X-ray at the turn of the century stands out as one of the most significant of the early scientific changes in the hospital, along with the establishment of diagnostic laboratories around the same time. Meanwhile, hospital research continued to be carried out by a few individual physicians, though even the larger hospitals did not accept or make much provision for research as a significant function of their institutions until the 1890s.

The historian Thomas McKeown argues that, for all such advances, even the best hospitals of the Western world did not play much of a role in reducing mortality until almost the end of this period, the late 1930s, when the sulfa drugs began to be available. Nevertheless, at the time they were introduced, the earlier improvements did help materially in improving the image of the hospital, at least in the American community. Above all, their introduction finally helped persuade the middle and upper classes of this country that the hospitals were indeed just as suitable for their own use as for the care of the poor. This revolution in attitudes did not take place overnight, but it was substantially completed by the 1930s. A particularly noteworthy aspect of the change was the steady acceptance by women of the upper classes, from early in the century, of the idea of moving childbirth to the hospital.

The various hospital improvements also gave medical practitioners added incentive to transfer the venue of their surgical operations, as well as the care of other seriously ill patients, from the home to the hospital. In communities with medical schools, the expanded patient populations in turn enhanced the use of the hospitals in teaching programs. This role was greatly extended, systematized, and strengthened after 1875. In fact, by the 1880s hospitals and medical schools were being planned and constructed side by side, as institutions with integrated activities and staffs and with enlarged facilities for scientific research. Following the examples furnished by the new Johns Hopkins medical institutions and a few other centers, the concept of the scientifically based teaching hospital took root in late-nineteenth-century America and spread rapidly in the next century. However, the new scientific character of the hospital was only one aspect of a widespread invigoration of medicine by science that took place during this period.

A Revolution in the Medical Sciences

Science, like the hospital, almost overnight came to assume a vastly altered and expanded position in the medical world of postbellum America. From the spare-time pursuit of a scattered few elite physicians, scientific research and related activities grew within a few decades into a huge biomedical enterprise involving thousands of highly trained specialists and technicians, many of them full time. From a mere handful of tiny facilities in the early 1870s—those at Ford's Theatre plus a scattering of pathological, chemical, and physiological laboratories—the institutions substantially involved in medical research mushroomed rapidly. By the 1920s, virtually every sizeable hospital, medical school, and health department, as well as every pharmaceutical company and relevant college science department, had its working laboratory. And in these facilities American scientists not only steadily increased their contributions to the fund of Western medical knowledge through research, but became involved on a large scale in such pursuits as the development of new diagnostic techniques, the delivery of analytic and diagnostic services, the production and testing of pharmaceutical and biological products, and the teaching of new physicians and medical scientists. While the lion's share of significant original discoveries, at least up to World War I, came from Europe, much of the direct application of the new knowledge to the health of mankind proved to be a predominantly American contribution.

The expansion of medical science in late-nineteenth- and early-twentieth-century America was accompanied and supported by the multiplication of such institutions as public libraries and museums, and even more directly by the reinvigoration and reshaping of the country's colleges and universities. It owed fully as much to the inventive genius, technologies, and profits associated with the nation's burgeoning industrial empire. But it derived its greatest force and immediacy from the increasing appreciation, adoption, and extension of the immensely significant contributions to medical knowledge that were then coming out of Europe.

Some American investigators set about to teach themselves the new European findings through the study of the published reports. And in this the large accumulations of literature in the Army Medical Library and other medical libraries played crucial roles. At the same time, however, more Americans than ever before decided that the best way to learn the intricacies of the modern scientific developments was by first-hand study under the European, particularly German, investigators for varying lengths of time.

The Americans particularly needed to learn the methods that had been so successful for the Europeans. This meant starting virtually from scratch to obtain an entirely new level of exposure to and familiarity with laboratories and with the equipment and procedures used in them. For, while a good many mid-nineteenth-century American medical practitioners had become adept at observational modes of research, few had much realization of the requirements, rigors, or challenges of laboratory work.

During the post–Civil War decades, therefore, a steadily growing wave of Americans made their way to medical and scientific institutions all over Europe, though particularly those in Germany, wherever the new laboratories had already produced notable results. For those interested in physiology, and in other medical sciences as well, the destination of choice at first was Carl Ludwig's famous laboratory at Leipzig, but additional laboratories and institutes quickly became attractive. Medical zoologists early had the choice of studying in such laboratories as those of Rudolf Leuckhardt or Raphael Blanchard or at the Zoological Station in Naples. Psychologists were increasingly attracted to Wilhelm Wundt's laboratory from the late 1870s onward. Hygiene could be studied at Max von Pettenkofer's Institute in Munich, pathology with such men as Rudolf Virchow in Berlin or Friedrich von Recklinghausen in Strasbourg. And, ultimately, the dramatic findings of bacteriology attracted Americans in large numbers to a variety of European laboratories, though above all to those of Robert Koch in Berlin and Louis Pasteur in Paris.

Following their European studies, these Americans came back to positions in colleges, universities, medical schools, and public health agencies. There they rapidly built up teaching programs in their respective scientific specialties and undertook their own research. Some prepared American textbooks on the new specialties. Others took the lead in creating societies, organizing journals, and otherwise strengthening and professionalizing their sciences.

Almost all took steps to build up their own laboratories, small and large. Many used their own money for this. Some, like William H. Welch at Johns Hopkins, received help from their universities, and others from government agencies. Still others, taking advantage of the age's emergent "Gospel of Wealth," successfully approached philanthropist-members of the new moneyed class. Louis Pasteur, painfully raising money for his own new institute and laboratories in Paris during the mid-1880s, regretted that he did not know any United States millionaires who might contribute. Benefactions from Andrew Carnegie and Cornelius Hoagland resulted in two excellent health laboratories—the Carnegie Laboratory and the Hoagland Laboratory—in the New York City area alone as early as the 1880s, while the even larger benefaction of John D. Rockefeller in 1903 created the Rockefeller Institute for Medical Research. Philanthropic contributions of the period also resulted in the establishment of several other research establishments, including the University of Pennsylvania's Institute of Hygiene and Chicago's McCormick Memorial Institute for Infectious Diseases.

From whatever source their funds came, by World War I the laboratories and scientific activities had emerged as not only essential but dominating features of the medical scene. They had become the key parts of what Daniel Fox has characterized as hierarchies of medical institutions and personnel in the various geographical regions, and through which the new medical and scientific knowledge was disseminated. Through such hierarchies American biomedical science, in the decades prior to 1940, was able to gain virtual parity with its European counterpart both in the extent of its institutions and services and in the general quality of its research.

Throughout this era, most of the scientific disciplines related to medicine changed substantially. The study of anatomy adapted in increasingly complex ways to the discoveries in physiology, pathology, and other sciences, but it retained much of its traditional importance at the center of medicine. Some of the other older health sciences and concerns, however, faded out of sight entirely or were altered almost beyond recognition. And in the process, in the United States as abroad, several new sciences emerged on the medical scene.

Physiologists, building on the pioneer mid-nineteenth-century contributions in their field, played central roles in reshaping American medicine through the post–Civil War period. An impressive number of them not only helped introduce experimental methods into various subareas of clinical research in this country, but went on to gain international reputations with their own research. Between 1900 and 1941, in fact, Americans made major contributions to almost every area of physiological research. Among these were Jacques Loeb in general physiology, Joseph Erlanger and Herbert Gasser in neurophysiology, and Walter Cannon in digestive and regulatory physiology. In their research, many of these investigators helped break down older barriers between the sciences even as they participated in shaping new specialties. Many physiologists, for instance, found themselves as deeply involved in chemistry as in traditional physiology. Ultimately, they organized themselves, as their European peers were doing, into the new professional and scientific entity of biochemistry, an entity which quickly acquired its own journals, societies, and other manifestations of a separate specialty.

By contrast with physiology, another of the older sciences, medical botany, gradually dropped virtually out of sight as the nineteenth century went on. Or rather, it was essentially abandoned by the medical regulars and left to certain of the sects. In any case, in the place of plant remedies, orthodox physicians, pharmacists, and chemists alike turned more and more to metallic substances and compounds. Late in the century, moreover, under the impact of experimental science, the familiar term *"materia medica"* steadily disappeared in favor of the new term, "pharmacology." Among the architects of this change was Johns Hopkins University's John Jacob Abel, the holder of America's first professorship of pharmacology. With their new knowledge and laboratory methods, Abel, his students, and other pharmacologists radically changed the study of drugs and their effects in the early-twentieth-century United States. And, in so doing, they contributed substantially to the processes of change in the field of pharmacy.

American pharmacy's overall development in the late nineteenth and early twentieth century continued parallel to that of orthodox medicine, though often independent of it. Further professional organization of the field was marked by a proliferation of state pharmaceutical associations during the 1870s and 1880s. During the same period, the small proprietary (for profit) colleges of pharmacy grew in number from thirteen in 1870 to fifty in 1900, but after that time the meager training provided by such institutions was rapidly replaced by full academic programs at many of the country's state universities, including extensive laboratory work in the sciences. Also during the last quarter of the nineteenth century, most states began the examination and licensure of pharmacists, while the federal government began the effective regulation of drug purity and safety in 1906.

Although professional pharmacists or druggists grew rapidly in number through this period, their technical roles as compounders of medicines often diminished. This was due largely to the increasingly easy availability in processed form of the various chemicals needed in medications, a trend which steadily did away with much of the process of preparing and compounding of drugs by the individual pharmacists. At the same time, the commercial side of their work increased, though it was often such sidelines as toiletries, hardware, groceries, or candies, along with soda fountains, which made the retail drugstores lucrative businesses.

Meanwhile, spurred by new technical processes and machines, American drug manufacturing companies also expanded considerably in size and number in the late nineteenth century. While some of these firms began establishing research facilities around 1900, in most cases research and development activities did not become prominent until World War I and the postwar period. The breakup of the German chemical cartel and the release of many of its key American patents at the latter time were particularly crucial in enabling the

American pharmaceutical industry to capture very large additional shares, not only of the United States business but of the international drug market.

During this period phrenology, while retaining some of its popular appeal, also declined as a serious area of orthodox scientific inquiry. Craniometry, likewise, though flourishing as a part of anthropology, progressively lost much of its interest for medical investigators. In place of phrenology and craniometry another science of mind gradually came into its own. Not illogically, the main part of the new science, psychology, had its origins in philosophy departments, where by the 1890s its adherents were installing laboratories and measuring mental behavior under controlled circumstances. American psychologists took the lead before World War I in testing reactions of industrial workers, while the Army went on, during that conflict, to test the intellectual capacities of recruits. These and other initiatives, particularly the further development of IQ tests, by 1940 had brought about a very broad application of psychological concepts and laboratory methods in many areas of American life. In the process, psychologists largely completed their split from philosophy and developed separate academic departments as well as created professional organizations and periodicals of their own. Many of its leaders, however—individuals such as Edward B. Titchener, John B. Watson, and Edwin Boring—tended to remain in the general university setting rather than to move into the medical schools.

Much like phrenology in the previous century, psychology did not remain an esoteric science of the professionals. On the contrary, its terms and concepts quickly achieved an enormous vogue among the general public as well. As such the activities of nonacademic popularizers and psychological testers became serious annoyances to the academicians and sometimes challenges to the integrity of psychology as an experimentally based science.

The introduction of psychoanalysis into American medical psychology was complicated by similar developments. Late-nineteenth-century psychiatry in the United States included few practitioners who were able to break away from the custodial preoccupations and constraints of the asylums. At the same time, the presence of numerous hospitalized Civil War veterans with severe nervous conditions provided an important impetus to the development of American neurology. S. Weir Mitchell, William A. Hammond, and other physicians made significant contributions at this time to the study and care of diseases and injuries of the nervous system. And several of them were active in bringing turn-of-the-century European psychiatric and psychological innovations to the attention of American professionals.

The Harvard neurologist James Jackson Putnam and the Clark University psychologist G. Stanley Hall were among those professionals who sponsored Sigmund Freud's trip to the United States in 1909 and who actively supported psychoanalysis. Despite much opposition, that measure gained adherents rapidly among medical doctors. These were physicians who used the new therapy extensively in the outpatient treatment of individuals suffering from neurotic conditions and to some extent even among the severely psychotic in mental hospitals. Beginning around the mid-1920s, psychoanalysis, the neurosciences, and clinical psychiatry all began to get important scientific recognition and research support from the Rockefeller philanthropies. However, during the same period psychoanalysis and other psychotherapies were often turned into medical fads among well-to-do patients as well as stylish topics for discussion at cocktail parties. Moreover, their concepts and terms became widely utilized by novelists and essayists, whose works in turn rapidly made them more or less familiar to many Americans.

Another of this country's changing scientific fields, that of heredity and genetics, was equally affected during this period by social considerations and imperatives. Mid-nineteenth-century interests in family and genealogy, as well as peoples' worries about the decline in vigor and number of the older white Anglo-Saxon Protestant stocks, carried over and were intensified after the Civil War. At the same time, earlier discussions about the origins and biological character of species and about race betterment were focused and directed into new experimental channels by various of the period's studies, not least of which were those of Charles Darwin. Studies of embryology, for one, were ultimately encouraged and expanded in this climate, as were investigations of the basic genetic character of animals, plants, and humans.

American laboratory research bearing on heredity was being done before 1896 by E. B. Wilson, while important genetics research along Mendelian lines was begun at Columbia University by Thomas Hunt Morgan around 1910. The development of human genetics, however, proved slow before 1940. This was due largely to the inhibitory effects of an expanding eugenics movement. Eugenicist concepts began to gain increased scientific sanction in the United States around the turn of the century under the influence of the works of England's Francis Galton, along with the introduction of statistical methods for analyzing the nature and distribution of hereditary traits, defects, and diseases. About the same time, eugenic marriage laws were passed in several states. Well before World War I, Charles Davenport and his Eugenic Record Office at Cold Spring Harbor, New York, became the focus of American research in the field and of the popular dissemination of increasingly racist information concerning it. American public opinion through the 1920s proved to be broadly responsive to this literature and supportive even of such extreme measures as sterilization of the feeble-minded at state institutions. Implementation of such measures in several American states was not missed by the following decade's social planners, physicians, and scientists in Nazi Germany.

Unlike genetics and some of the other sciences, the late nineteenth-century development of pathology, the science of disease, was not divided or seriously diverted by essentially social or popular considerations. During the middle decades of the nineteenth century, in the United States as abroad, the science became increasingly precise in elucidating the nature of disease. Particularly influential in this was the German scientist Rudolf Virchow's concept of cellular pathology as it developed within the framework of the expanding physiological knowledge. Throughout these decades, however, answers to the ultimate questions about the causation of diseases, particularly infectious diseases, continued to elude pathologists. For some, contagionist theories of disease were increasingly bolstered by laboratory findings obtained by ever more powerful microscopes. But anticontagionist or environmentalist concepts of the same period were almost equally supported by field observations of facts in such sciences as climatology, medical topography and epidemiology, some of them fields that had their own sophisticated instruments though they were lacking in effective controls.

The proofs of the germ theory of disease causation which were advanced by Koch, Pasteur, and their followers in the decades after 1870 did not drive the environmental concepts out of medical thinking overnight. But they did provide an ultimately persuasive demonstration of the importance of the laboratory in medical research. In fact, by the end of the nineteenth century some of the new branches of experimental pathology—notably bacteriology and its offshoot, immunology—had become, in America as well as in Europe, among the most prestigious and appealing of the new medical sciences. In the process, medical climatology and topography, along with epidemiology, dropped out of medical fashion for the next several decades.

The American phase of the age of bacteriology was launched on a small scale by scattered scientists in the early 1880s at a few university and governmental laboratories. But the adoption of bacteriological methods did not become at all widespread for another decade and more. The army physician George Sternberg published a text on bacteriology as early as 1892, while journals, societies, and other paraphernalia of professionalism were appearing by 1900. American investigators often began their research in the field by replicating the early European studies of bacteria. However, such experiments soon expanded to include other kinds of disease-causing organisms as well, to study the vast, largely-microscopic worlds of helminths, protozoa, insects, and viruses. Thus, by the 1890s, Sternberg had independently discovered the pneumococcus, while William H. Welch had identified the causative bacillus of gas gangrene. In 1893, moreover, Theobald Smith and his colleagues in the United States Department of Agriculture announced their important discovery of the role of ticks in the transmission of Texas cattle fever. Within a few years Americans had also made significant contributions to unraveling the relationships of parasites to hookworm disease, yellow fever, and Rocky Mountain spotted fever. Other investigators became productively engaged in research on the applied aspects of immunology, standardization of the production of vaccines or sera used in rabies, smallpox, diphtheria, typhoid, and other diseases, and the improvement of methods of storing and using them. A number of so-called "Pasteur Institutes" were formed in the United States late in the nineteenth century mainly to produce these and other biological products. But within a few years much of this kind of business had been taken over by the commercial drug industry as an adjunct of its own increasing research activities.

From its founding and throughout the early decades of the twentieth century the focal point of much of America's fundamental research in bacteriology was the Rockefeller Institute. Scientists of the first rank—individuals such as Simon Flexner and Hideyo Noguchi—conducted ever more sophisticated studies there on the various infectious diseases. And, like scientists at other institutions, they made progressively more significant contributions to immunology and other sciences. In the process, the Institute gained professional recognition as the country's premier medical research center. By the 1930s, moreover, thanks largely to such writers as Paul de Kruif and Sinclair Lewis, it had become familiar to the general public. As such, for many Americans the Institute stood out as the most conspicuous symbol of the twentieth-century's new laboratory-oriented medicine.

The membership of the period's medical profession was not by any means of a single mind about the desirability of bringing the various findings and methods of laboratory science rapidly into the practical world of medicine. Many sectarian physicians found it difficult to see, at first anyway, how the new concepts could fit into their systems. Moreover, the concepts and findings meant little or nothing to considerable numbers of regular practitioners as well. These included doctors who had received their training in inferior medical schools; some whose local medical libraries still had few of the late books or journals; others who were reasonably content using the simple *materia medica* of their fathers; and yet others who had had little or no experience with microscopes in their practices and who had little basis for understanding the laboratory environment or the research mentality.

Many practitioners were simply indifferent to the new science as something which was outside their ken. Some, however, were more or less hostile to its implications or methods. One segment of these, who had made respectable contributions to environmental or observational sciences, were understandably resentful on being told that those sciences were suddenly obsolete. Another large group well into the twentieth century remained unconvinced by the claimed proofs of the germ theory of disease. And still others continued to feel that laboratory investigations involving animal experimentation were immoral.

Whatever the numbers of the doubters and objectors, the enthusiasts rapidly became more vocal and more influential in pressing their arguments for large new roles for science in medicine. To begin with anyway, the most avid enthusiasts came primarily from among the best-educated and well-to-do physicians, individuals already committed to the improvement of medicine and with the means of continuing that pursuit. Members of this elite went to great pains, through long hours of study in the medical libraries as well as during their trips to Europe, to make themselves familiar with the new knowledge and methods. And, having done so, many of them, of whom Welch was a conspicuous example, went on to influential medical positions as professors, deans, health officers, and editors. Through such leadership positions they effectively guided the bulk of the new generation of physicians to an acceptance of the new science as an essential central element, not only in hospitals, medical schools, and public health procedures, but in everyday practice.

This is not to say that very many of the exciting research developments of the early age of bacteriology and pharmacology were transformed at all rapidly into therapies that could help the practitioner deal with his patients' diseases. In any case, not a few late-nineteenth-century doctors were still guided to some extent by the therapeutic skepticism of their forefathers. Reflecting that, the practice of bleeding continued to decline, though some physicians still kept leeches on hand. Moreover, the practitioner already had a number of familiar and significant drugs at his disposal. Mercury, morphine, opium, quinine, and digitalis, among others, had come down from earlier generations, while during the nineteenth century such drugs as ether, cocaine, aspirin, codeine, and iodine came into use. Late in the nineteenth century, the administration of sera and vaccines also became a steadily more significant part of orthodox therapeutics, no longer just for smallpox but now for rabies, diphtheria, typhoid, and other diseases. Subsequently, a few highly effective drugs also emerged from the new laboratories, sometimes to the accompaniment of exuberant public acclaim. These included salvarsan and adrenalin before World War I, insulin in the 1920s, and the sulfa drugs in the late 1930s, each of them stirring up hopes that additional remarkable medications were not far behind.

New Strengths and Configurations of Mainline Medicine

The post–Civil War development of America's medical profession was less dramatic and represented somewhat less of a break with the past than did that of the medically related sciences. Still, modifications during this period were substantial and far-reaching. Building on the momentum of changes that had already begun, as well as on the contributions of the sciences, the organized "regular" profession added immeasurably to its strength and effectiveness. In the process, its authority and public standing at the head of an enlarged medical establishment was substantially advanced, although that primacy was by no means universally acknowledged.

The centennial year of 1876 provided an occasion for some of the regulars to reflect on the status and achievements of mainline medicine since the Revolution. Focusing on the contributions to "practical" medicine and surgery of the country's medical elite—a small coterie of well-trained physicians who would have been a credit to any country—the physician-historians seemed generally well pleased by the record of results. If no American Galen or Harvey or Paracelsus had as yet turned up, the relatively modest initiatives of this native elite had nevertheless enabled medicine to keep "steady pace with the general progress of the arts and sciences on this continent" through the nineteenth century. All in all, they concluded, given America's circumstances as a new nation, "we have no reason [either] to boast, or to be ashamed of what we have thus far accomplished."

The authors did not pretend that America's ordinary medicine matched Europe's best. Nor did they pay much attention to any of the country's medical shortcomings or problems. There was little ref-

erence to the sectarian beliefs and practices that still challenged mainline medicine. They said nothing about the abysmally poor qualifications of a considerable proportion of the regulars. Moreover, they
hardly mentioned the substantial shortages of universities, hospitals,
laboratories, and other resources that had to be alleviated before
American medicine could either meet the pressing social needs or
match the more advanced European levels.

The late-nineteenth-century orthodox profession did indeed have
a sizeable agenda, though in many respects it differed little from
that of the antebellum period. Regular physicians still focused their
collective energies heavily on such basic matters as the battle against
the irregular sects, the campaigns to obtain effective medical licensing
legislation, the struggle against quackery, the urgent need to elevate
the quality of medical education, and the equally pressing need to
improve America's contributions to medical literature. However, neither the nature nor the magnitude of these problems was the same
as it had been. Above all, they seemed somehow to have become far
less intractable than before. By World War I, in fact, regular physicians could point to substantial betterment in almost every phase of
their professional lives.

Central to much of this change, and virtually unbelievable to almost all concerned, was the gradual post–Civil War emergence of a
rapprochement between regular practitioners and those belonging
to the surviving major medical sects, homeopathy and eclecticism.
Leaders on both sides slowly began to admit, at least to themselves,
in the 1870s and 1880s, that their respective modes of practice had
been steadily losing many of their points of difference. Besides, no-
body had been benefiting very much from the ongoing medical hostilities. Orthodox practitioners came to realize that their attacks on the
sectarians actually tended to make the latter stronger. It was increasingly apparent to the regulars, moreover, given the public's continuing endorsement of medical pluralism, that new medical licensing
laws could not be pushed through the various state legislatures so
long as they discriminated against the sects. At the same time, specialists in the larger cities, most of whom were orthodox doctors,
were increasingly aware that patient referrals from sectarian general
practitioners could become lucrative parts of their own practices, but
this could only come about if orthodox codes of ethics were modified
or relaxed.

For their part, not a few sectarian physicians perceived that key
therapeutic principles of their sects were fast becoming untenable. A
growing number had begun to use the standard therapies of the

regulars. Many irregulars saw that their separatist positions too often barred them from desirable roles in the various community medical institutions, particularly hospitals.

While many regulars consistently resisted conceding anything to sectarianism, others in the profession made the period between 1870 and 1915 a time of increasing medical compromise and accommodation. In one community after another, orthodox physicians tired of their fruitless fights against the sectarians and hesitantly allowed themselves to be drawn into certain professional contacts with old foes. Prominently, they were forced by circumstances to collaborate with the latter in working out licensing laws that would benefit both sides against the unorganized "quacks." They soon found themselves serving with sectarian doctors on public medical examining boards. Along the way, regulars came to realize that many homeopaths and eclectics were as well trained as they were, and they slowly relaxed their rules against consulting with such practitioners.

Formal acceptance of the sectarians, however, did not come until after the turn of the century. In a climactic move, the American Medical Association in 1903 finally removed most of the long-standing strictures against sectarianism from its code of ethics. And, within a short time, orthodox medical institutions began opening their doors to well-qualified practitioners of the older sects.

While the regulars were uneasily making contacts possible, the concerned sects, the homeopaths and eclectics, at first continued their successful fight for legal sanction. They also added to the numbers of their medical schools and hospitals and generally continued to flourish. However, the important objective for most of their practitioners, as Paul Starr has emphasized, seems to have been the gaining of professional acceptance from the regulars. Accordingly, when that finally came about, at the turn of the century, with its attendant access to the privileges of the regulars, the main reason for continuing their separate identities as homeopaths and eclectics began to dissolve. Large numbers of these former sectarians thereupon rapidly came to think of themselves as part of the medical mainstream. As this number increased, the professional paraphernalia of the two sects—their medical schools, societies, and hospitals—began an amazingly rapid process of withering away or of changing their identities from sectarian to regular bodies. By the 1930s the process was virtually complete, leaving only a handful of homeopathic practitioners and an occasional homeopathic drugstore on the fringes of the medical world.

Even as American mainline medicine was being relieved of the longstanding incubus of its enervating hostilities between regulars and the older sects, it was being further strengthened and animated by very substantial improvements in the quality of the training received by physicians. The elevation of medical education had been high on the reform agendas of medical leaders, at least since the 1840s. But improvements had been frustratingly few and slow in coming. Throughout the century, though some competent practitioners regularly emerged from the system, in general the American proprietary schools, with their meager facilities and notoriously low standards, continued to churn out large numbers of grossly unprepared medical doctors. Moreover, even less reputable late-nineteenth-century diploma mills, for a fee, supplied credentials through the mails.

The post–Civil War period, however, also brought various changes for the better. Among these were modifications introduced as part of the general rejuvenation of American higher education of that period. At Harvard University, prominently, the reforms of President Charles W. Eliot in the 1870s included bringing the virtually autonomous medical school, over the bitter objections of the medical faculty, under the umbrella of effective university control. Subsequently, over the next several decades, Harvard and other institutions proceeded to elevate the quality of their medical instruction through such basic steps as raising admissions qualifications, lengthening academic terms, building up laboratory and other facilities, and expanding curricula. A few of the new medical schools of the 1880s and 1890s incorporated such changes from the outset, and some went on to still other innovations, such as Johns Hopkins University's controversial requirement that its medical faculty be full time. Many of these were changes that were strongly urged by physicians returning from their studies in European universities. And the way to their adoption was eased by the wider ferments in science education and research that were going on in many of the institutions that had affiliated medical schools.

By 1910 the leaders of the American medical community had given these matters much attention and had formed a firm idea of what they thought all of the country's medical schools should become. In the Johns Hopkins school as it had developed under Welch and his colleagues, they had what amounted to a prototype. But it was well known that there still were hardly more than half a dozen other institutions that came close to measuring up to the Hopkins standard. Just how poor many of the remainder still were was disclosed that year in a notable report prepared by the educator Abraham Flexner for the Carnegie Foundation for the Advancement of Teaching. Flexner's report was based upon personal visits to 157 medical schools in the United States and 8 in Canada, and including sectarian as well as regular institutions. In it, Flexner included short factual summaries and evaluations of each school with respect to five criteria: entrance requirements, size of teaching staffs, financial status, laboratory facilities, and clinical resources.

The publication and wide circulation of Flexner's report gave a notable boost to the ongoing reform efforts within the individual institutions, as well as within the American Medical Association, the Association of American Medical Colleges, and other segments of the medical profession. It had the immediate effect of finally pressuring a large number of the country's weaker medical schools out of existence within a remarkably short period, including a considerable proportion of the remaining sectarian medical schools. For many leaders of these institutions, closure was predominantly determined by the economics of the situation. It was a step forced upon them by the prohibitively expensive costs of laboratories and clinical facilities that they now saw they would need in order to continue to compete.

By the World War I period, this sharp decline in the number of schools brought about a rapid reduction in the production of new physicians, along with a sharp increase in competition among candidates for admission to the surviving medical schools. In order to survive and compete, the remaining schools now felt compelled to discontinue their proprietary character, to strengthen their links with hospitals and universities, and generally to elevate their standards and improve their facilities still further. To advance this process, some of the higher-ranked schools were singled out to receive substantial foundation assistance. Such awards ultimately enabled these institutions to emerge, in the 1920s and 1930s, as elite centers of medical excellence, centers in which the pursuit of research eventually came to be as prominent as the production of medical practitioners.

Important agencies in much of the reform in medical education, as well as in other aspects of professional change among the regulars, were the medical societies. True, through the end of the nineteenth century, the regular societies were relatively weak, poorly organized, and not particularly representative bodies. As late as 1900, the American Medical Association had only 8,000 members, less than 7 percent of the nation's physicians. Fewer than a third even belonged to a state or local society. Those who were members, however, sometimes managed to steer their societies into active postbellum involvement in medical school reform. Society members and committees also played central roles in obtaining new state licensing legislation. And the society meetings were the critical arenas where the new concessions to homeopaths and eclectics were painfully worked out. Nevertheless, throughout the nineteenth century, the medical societies were notorious for their general ineffectiveness in representing the interests of their members.

This changed rapidly after 1901. In that year the American Medical Association was reorganized as the keystone of a confederation of state and local societies. This organizational overhaul enhanced the standing and effectiveness of the societies at all levels of the hierarchy. And it had the immediate effect of drawing large numbers of previously unaffiliated physicians to the societies as new members.

Medical society revenues went up along with memberships. These resources permitted the societies to engage paid staffs and to expand their activities. Many of the state societies, for instance, began publishing their own professional journals at this time. This trend was part of a more general burgeoning of America's medically related journals of all stripes, an expansion that tripled the ninety-four periodicals of 1878 within about three decades. The American Medical Association, with its own new journal as well as its new funds and an aggressive secretariat, became increasingly involved and influential in various matters after 1901. It played a leading role in food and drug reform. It pursued the war against quacks with ever greater energy. It demonstrated a new interest in public health matters with such activities as its push for a federal department of health and its sponsorship in 1914 of a nationwide survey of state health departments. Moreover, around the same time, if only briefly, its committees were even exploring the merits of national health insurance.

By the 1920s and 1930s, the American Medical Association, acting nationally for the local societies, was exerting a degree of power in shaping the direction and content of public medical policy that had been previously undreamed of. While by no means speaking for all health interests, it was nevertheless acknowledged as being by far the strongest of America's medical interest groups. Moreover, it quickly achieved a place in most people's minds, for good or bad, as the increasingly conservative embodiment of the nation's medical establishment.

With the various changes, orthodox physicians came to enjoy a steadily improving status and authority. While few of them, outside of specialists, seem to have gained noticeably larger incomes, nonetheless a new degree of self-assurance spread throughout the profession, a trait that opponents or outsiders sometimes saw as arrogance. In their local society meetings, individual physicians gradually shed much of their defensiveness and pessimism. And, as science began to produce more knowledge that physicians could agree about, together with additional effective therapies, the meetings also lost much of the futile acrimony that had helped keep the profession so divided during the nineteenth century.

Conspicuous as symbols of the new well-being and power of the profession, especially in Philadelphia, Boston, New York, and other large cities, were the increasingly large, and sometimes sumptuous, buildings erected by the medical societies. These edifices housed the societies' meeting rooms, administrative offices, portraits of eminent doctors, and sometimes collections of medical artifacts. In many cases, the interiors were dominated by the richly panelled reading rooms of the society libraries. Well before this period not a few societies, as well as hospitals and medical schools, maintained libraries, generally modest at best. During the early and mid-nineteenth century, however, well-to-do physicians amassed large libraries, personal holdings which included not only the current professional literature but impressive collections of rare medical works. Eventually many of these collections were sold or given away, frequently to the medical society libraries, sometimes to libraries connected with medical schools. For some prominent turn-of-the-century physicians, among them William H. Welch and William Osler, the study of these libraries' holdings of classic works, the productions of the great doctors of past ages, offered a much-needed humanistic perspective for a profession caught up in modern experimental medicine. The interests of most of the period's doctors, however, tended to be confined to the libraries' rapidly proliferating holdings of the current medical literature, for these were the books and journals which had to be studied in order to understand and keep up with the period's explosion of medical science.

Meanwhile, around the turn of the century, the doctor's day-to-day activity was being modified by innovations growing out of science and technology. Physicians came under increasing pressure to wash their hands and sterilize their instruments before touching their patients. Health departments enlarged their demands on them to report their cases of infectious diseases. Steadily improved diagnostic devices became available: thermometers and stethoscopes finally came into wide use; eye charts, spirometers, and blood pressure devices appeared at physical examinations; endoscopes, laryngoscopes and other instruments increased the capacity to look into the interior of the body. At the same time, physicians steadily tranferred more of their operations to hospitals, where even more elaborate instruments and items of equipment were becoming available. And, not least, the services of laboratories became progressively more essential to the practitioners for doing X-rays or making diagnostic tests of stools, urine, blood, and sputum.

These and other innovations helped make for substantial changes in the atmosphere around and conditions at the late-nineteenth- and early-twentieth-century sickbed. The spread of anesthesia by itself continued to greatly reduce the patient's fears of painful operations, while prescriptions of narcotics made the pains from nonoperable conditions more bearable. Meanwhile, bolstered by better training, new instruments, laboratory aids to diagnosis, and improved medications, physicians steadily lost much of their age-old uncertainty at the bedside.

The care and support provided by the family circle itself remained crucially important to the general well-being and morale of the seriously ill or dying person in America, but some of the family's traditional roles gradually diminished during this period. A major factor in bringing this about was the shifting of the locale of much medical care, both of the poor and the well-to-do, from the home to the hospital, with its greater concentrations of medical equipment, services, and personnel. The bedside attendants now became predominantly professionals—nurses, physicians, technicians—rather than family members. Moreover, as the twentieth century went on, the well-to-do hospital patient could also demand telephones, radios, library services, and other amenities. The poor patient, in place of such comforts, often found his privacy invaded by medical professors teaching their classes at the bedside.

In and out of the hospitals, the knowledge and appurtenances of modern laboratory medicine gradually brought new hope and comfort to seriously ill persons and their families. Fewer (or different) fears and reservations came to be expressed about either the surgical interventions or the medical regimens proposed by their physicians. And as people gained more confidence in medical measures, their direct reliance upon religious measures and faith tended to lessen. Nevertheless, a great many of America's sick or their families regularly continued to ask for visits from family ministers or hospital chaplains. Clerical prayers and other supports remained particularly important parts of the personal preparation of the dying. However, the clergy less often encountered the attending physicians on these occasions; for many members of the medical profession, the care of the soul and concern for the afterlife had come to have little to do with the problems of managing illness.

Most physicians of the half-century or so following the Civil War continued to act and be identified as general practitioners. However, the proliferation of biological and medical knowledge was increasingly conducive to medical specialization. Particularly in large cities, more and more general practitioners turned themselves into specialists and even subspecialists in such fields as anesthesiology, internal medicine, ophthalmology, and dermatology. Dentists eventually often narrowed their practice to areas such as orthodontics, while many nurses developed specialized practices in industries, schools, or other clienteles. At the same time, the specialties refined their techniques and built up their professional paraphernalia of societies, journals, and eventually, specialty examining boards. As one example of this evolution, the superintendents of "insane asylums" gradually acquired new professional identities as psychiatrists. Surgeons, meanwhile, rapidly divided themselves into subspecialties and often, as in the cases of William S. Halsted, Harvey Cushing, and Alexis Carrel, built up distinctive and formidable mystiques in the process. However, it was perhaps the obstetricians who best epitomized the new strength of specialties with their twentieth-century successes in driving most of the remaining midwives out of business or underground, transferring most deliveries from the home to the hospital, and otherwise virtually completing the "medicalization" of childbirth.

The pursuits of specialists as well as general practitioners in post–Civil War America, including the regulars' activities in their professional organizations and in health care institutions, continued to be predominantly a world of white males. Both women and blacks became more numerous in the profession, but at least through World War II their involvement was sharply limited by prevailing social prejudices. Women, following the Civil War, established several additional separate medical schools for women, along with a few special hospitals in which women physicians could practice. Late in the century, some of the regular medical schools finally became effectively coeducational, a development which ultimately led to the disappearance of the separate womens' schools. However, the regular medical societies remained notoriously conservative in this respect even longer. The American Medical Association did not admit women until 1915 and some other bodies even later.

Under such inhibitions, the proportion of American physicians who were women remained small. Up to 1940 the number of women among the graduates of indigenous medical schools never rose above 6 percent of the total. At the same time, however, as Starr points out, during the twentieth century well-trained women were increasingly employed as technical assistants in hospital laboratories and other departments where they offered little challenge to the authority or economic position of the male doctors.

Blacks under freedom were even more thoroughly barred from the post–Civil War medical establishment than were women. They were unable to obtain membership in the regular medical societies and were effectively excluded from most hospital staffs throughout this period. As a consequence, they were forced to develop what amounted to a virtually complete separate medical establishment and medical care system of their own parallel to that of the whites. The formalization of separate medical education for blacks began with the opening of the Howard University Medical Department in 1868, with assistance from the United States Freedmen's Bureau. Meharry Medical College, founded by the Methodist Church, emerged in 1876, followed by other black schools, many of them short-lived. While seven still existed at the time of Flexner's survey, only Howard and Meharry survived that experience and continued to the 1980s. Meanwhile, black physicians began organizing their own local societies as early as 1870. A broader-based group, the National Medical Association, was created in 1895, while separate medical journals run by and for black physicians also began to appear in the 1890s.

The organization of separate hospitals for blacks was an equally important step, since most of the age's new hospitals either refused outright to accept blacks as patients or gave them highly inferior accommodations and care. By 1910 some hundred black hospitals had come into existence, virtually the only medical care institutions where black physicians could practice or obtain clinical training. However, the ratio of trained black physicians to the country's black population remained highly inadequate throughout this period. And with only these limited opportunities for training, together with the rising costs of medical education, the numbers of black medical graduates actually declined steadily year by year. Given the social and economic conditions, the separate medical establishment of the blacks thus could only mitigate and never fully meet the desperate medical situation of blacks in pre-1940 America.

Social discrimination also had its effects on the access of other segments of America's population to mainline medical institutions and services. Catholics, who began erecting their own hospitals during the antebellum period as part of their effort to survive in a Protestant society, had accumulated over 150 such institutions by 1885. They also supported a medical school (Georgetown) as early as 1851 and added several others early in the twentieth century. Catholics continued to encounter discrimination well into the twentieth century in their applications for admission to non-Catholic medical schools, as well as in their candidacies for hospital internships or residencies. Scattered separate Jewish hospitals were organized during the nineteenth century and considerably more during the twentieth century. Discrimination against Jewish applicants for medical school admission actually increased after 1900, when the success of such candidates became so great as to seem threatening to the dominant WASP medical community. After World War I, in fact, many medical schools, along with other institutions of higher education, introduced quotas on the numbers of Jews accepted, a practice that continued into mid-century.

The medicine that was practiced by a majority of the Catholic and Jewish physicians during this period, as well as by America's women and blacks, among their respective clienteles, undoubtedly differed little from the therapeutics of the male white Anglo-Saxon Protestant practitioners. However, the systematic exclusion of such physicians from the medical establishment and its institutions effectively belied any pretension that the establishment could, during the late-nineteenth- and early-twentieth-century decades, speak as the unquestioned voice of American medicine. The force of such claims was also brought into question by the rise of new formal medical sects, and even more by the expanding character of other far-flung health-related activities, most of them with little or no connection with the interests and pursuits of mainline medical practitioners.

Continuing Health Pursuits outside the Establishment

Despite the new strengths of mainline medicine, nonestablishment health-related groups or movements did not by any means wither away. In fact, America's tradition of medical diversity continued and even took on new dimensions and strengths of its own in the age of scientific medicine. As in earlier generations, this diversity grew partly out of Americans' habits of self-medication and their clinging to the right of medical choice. However, it gained a more timely modern character with the gathering of movements or organizations that reflected people's consciousness of new threats to personal health and well-being, as well as of health needs that so far were not being met.

The flourishing of medical diversity between 1865 and 1940 continued to owe a great deal to the limited scope of regular medicine. For all its new hospitals, instruments, learning, and status, mainline medicine still did not go very far in treating certain kinds of maladies.

And above all it was little involved in the various areas of hygiene. Laypeople were well aware that most regular physicians were neither interested in nor trained to deal with hygienic concerns and often considered them unimportant. In fact, the regulars consistently seemed to ignore any health-related matters that failed to fit in with the objectives, values, and institutions of modern scientific medicine.

For their part, individual post–Civil War Americans gradually gained more confidence in medical doctors than previous generations had had, and they utilized their services to a commensurately greater extent. Certainly, some of the old suspicions that people had harbored about the educated physician began to dissipate during this period. At the same time, however, relatively few people relied entirely on any one kind of practitioner or therapy alone for all of their medical care.

Most ordinary citizens, in fact, continued to take care of many of their illnesses by themselves. They dealt with many or most of their own everyday injuries, fevers, stomach aches, bites, and other complaints, along with those of their family members. They continued to rely on old family recipes as well as on home treatment manuals and almanacs. Health advice literature of all kinds continued to be an extremely popular consumer product.

To an even greater extent, Americans were also consumers of bandages and other kinds of medical supplies, but above all, of medications of every sort. Their voracious demand for these items ensured the multiplication of drugstores and the continued growth of legitimate drug manufacturers. It also guaranteed that the country's patent medicine makers and vendors of alleged "quack" remedies of all kinds would remain numerous and often prosperous well into the twentieth century, even in the face of repeated efforts to regulate them out of existence. As part of this, American citizens of all classes were increasingly bombarded, during the decades after the Civil War, by advertisements in the press and in new mass audience periodicals for such remedies and treatments. After World War I, radio also came into effective use. While spokespersons for medical as well as lay groups expressed alarm over the widespread ballyhooing of these remedies, many Americans proved receptive to such advertising and, if one remedy failed to give relief, they were generally ready to try another.

Late-nineteenth- and early-twentieth-century news accounts of the various laboratory breakthroughs brought more complicated reader responses. Much popular interest was aroused in the United States by dispatches providing details of Pasteur's dramatic early serum treatments of rabies victims, Koch's claims of a cure for tuberculosis, and the release of Ehrlich's "magic bullet" for syphilis, among other discoveries. In the United States as elsewhere, such developments stirred up hope that cures for every kind of disease were imminent. However, as long as the ordinary regular physicians proved unable to meet such expectations, not a few of their patients fell back once again to a reliance on the patent medicines and quack remedies. At the same time, Americans were far from being entirely comfortable with the changes taking place in medicine. For many, the new items of equipment in the doctors' offices and hospitals were more fearsome than assuring. The entire world of laboratory medicine, in fact, frequently seemed alien to layperson. Its basic fund of knowledge was esoteric and beyond the understanding of all but the well educated, while the rationale for its experimental procedures was not evident. Above all, for not a few, laboratory medicine appeared as a threat to certain cherished values. These fears led to several organized turn-of-the-century protest movements.

Serious and thoughtful resistance to animal experimentation began to be noticeable in the United States during the relatively early phases of modern scientific medicine. Localized antivivisection sentiment appeared in New York City during the late 1860s in protest against animal experimentation that was being carried out by the physicians John C. Dalton and Austin Flint, Jr. In New York and other cities, such sentiment centered originally in the newly formed humane societies and antivivisection societies, but it subsequently spread through other, notably upper-class, groups. As physiological and bacteriological laboratories continued to proliferate around the country later in the century, the protests against animal experiments multiplied correspondingly, and a spate of proposals for restrictive legislation were aired. Some of these resulted, during the 1890s, in local laws that placed limits on animal experiments. However, efforts to outlaw such experimentation entirely were easily defeated by the concentrated efforts of America's medical and scientific leaders. This early phase of antivivisection sentiment then quickly lost most of its momentum, and by World War I the movement had dwindled to a handful of overt supporters.

Organized public protests also arose, at least briefly during the 1890s, against the adoption of diphtheria antitoxin. Likewise, around the same period, resistance to smallpox vaccination flared up anew in certain cities, sometimes violently, as health officials tried to enforce its use among immigrant populations. Comparable, if less violent, reactions surfaced after World War II in various communities when officials began considering the addition of fluorides to public water supplies as a measure to reduce dental caries.

Another demonstration of people's reservations about mainline medicine was their continuing support for more or less organized therapeutic movements or sects. One of the remarkable medical phenomena of the *fin-de-siècle* period was the failure of the regular medical establishment, despite its new strength, to prevent the emergence of new sects, rising as they did in some cases phoenixlike virtually from the ashes of the old. These new sects did not collectively gain the same degree of therapeutic importance that homeopathy, botanical medicine, eclecticism, and hydropathy had occupied during the nineteenth century. However, they came to play far more than token roles in fostering a continuing skepticism of, if not actual resistance to, orthodox medical authority. Dealing as they did with illness and pain in ways that differed from the scientific medicine of the regulars, they provided society with a new set of medical options.

Some of these post–Civil War movements grew out of a new involvement of clergymen and other religiously motivated individuals in therapy. The need that had existed in earlier generations for America's clergymen to fill in as medical practitioners had virtually ended well before the Civil War. However, the late nineteenth century saw various clergymen and laymen attempting to reclaim a certain portion of this role, particularly through faith healing or religious mental therapy. At least partly because of the lack of interest in such matters on the part of most trained physicians, two of the groups that were organized to provide such therapies became particularly substantial and significant.

Christian Science took shape in the 1870s in New England, with the publication by Mary Baker Eddy of her basic teachings, *Science and Health*, and the organization of the first congregations. Over the next several decades, the group became nationwide in scope with the formation of teaching facilities and publications, together with the creation of numerous other congregations, nearly 500 by 1900. With its roots in phrenology, mesmerism, and homeopathy, as well as in Christianity, Christian Science was a form of mind cure whose appeal lay in its frank repudiation of traditional concepts of disease and of mainline medicine's materialistic therapeutics. As such, it quickly gained the hostility of organized medicine as a result of the well-publicized claims of cures effected by its practitioners as well as because of the church's considerable success around the country in gaining exemption for those practitioners from medical licensing laws.

The Christian Science movement was early criticized for its upper-class orientation and its neglect of the needs of the poor, including their health needs. At the same time, the considerable popularity of Eddy's teachings suggested to others that there might be a further place for religious therapeutics, even within the established denominations. One particularly significant result was the Emmanuel Movement, which developed within Boston's Emmanuel Church (Episcopal) soon after 1900. The minister of the church, Elwood Worcester, was not only deeply committed to current social gospel ideals but familiar both with modern experimental psychology and psychotherapeutic concepts. With the support and participation of prominent Boston physicians and others, Worcester organized a three-fold community program in his church that included clinical care, health education, and psychotherapeutic counseling. As conducted in Boston over the next several decades, this movement, too, gained the hostility of organized medicine. Nevertheless, its therapeutic features spread widely through America's Protestant denominations, furnishing important models for subsequent pastoral psychology.

Of the other new therapeutic movements, most focused upon aspects of people's physical health that the regular physicians conspicuously neglected. Osteopathy, a native American movement founded by Andrew T. Still late in the nineteenth century, was designed to relieve pain and restore health broadly through manipulations and restorations of the body's structural components. The earliest osteopathic schools and infirmaries were founded in the Midwest during the 1890s and were followed by similar institutions elsewhere, along with professional journals and associations. Osteopaths were licensed to practice in a few states even before 1900, and in around twenty by 1920. By 1940 there were some 8,000 such practitioners. In fact, the sect gained steadily not only in numbers but in popularity and in respectability. Gradually incorporating many features of regular medicine into their original system of treatment, by World War II most osteopaths were functioning much like regular physicians.

Chiropractic, likewise introduced in the late 1890s, also aimed to provide relief through manipulative methods. The brainchild of another midwesterner, Daniel D. Palmer, chiropractic treatment focused on the spine and nervous system. While the sect did not increase as rapidly as osteopathy, it nevertheless could claim as many as seventy-nine of its own schools by 1920, together with various societies and journals, while by 1930 it included over 16,000 practitioners. However, chiropractors were far less inclined than osteopathists to compromise their fundamental approach to therapy. Accordingly, the orthodox medical establishment persistently pictured chiropractic to the public as a particularly unsavory form of quackery.

Partly due to this, the movement gained little political support during this period and was licensed in comparatively few states.

Among other new medical movements that rose early in the twentieth century was optometry. In this case, some of the initiative came from opticians interested in expanding the commercial scope of their trade. But major encouragement came from members of the public who found that physicians were generally poorly prepared to prescribe for peoples' needs for glasses. Even fewer doctors—one in forty-five as late as 1909—had training in eye refraction. As opticians converted themselves into optometrists, or at least began using that name, the public proved increasingly happy to patronize them. For, as optometrists, they not only provided eyeglass frames and lenses but the necessary diagnosis, refraction, and prescription as well, all at a lower price than if the patient had to go through the medical profession. Despite opposition from medical regulars, particularly the ophthalmologists, optometrists rapidly organized themselves under this new name and by 1917 had succeeded in obtaining legislative sanction in all but a few of the American states.

Even more extended in size and scope than the new formal therapies or sects were those movements and groups that were devoted to the improvement of personal health. In fact, many of the familiar concepts and practices of hygiene took on new shapes in the sociomedical ferment of the post–Civil War decades. Some individuals continued to bring forward comprehensive regimens aimed generally at warding off ill health and promoting long life. Others focused on ways of offsetting or combating specific hygienic ills. Certain of their enterprises relied to a considerable extent on the findings of modern science, but most of them focused above all on promoting hygienic self-discipline and on utilizing the healing resources of nature. As such they constituted nuclei of support for the age's vigorous pursuit of the Spencerian ideal of the survival of the fittest.

While health professionals contributed to the success of some of these enterprises, for the most part the medical doctors remained notoriously uninterested in disease prevention. As a result, the multifaceted health enterprise remained a predominantly lay initiative. Nevertheless, its scale was little if any less than that of organized medicine in the numbers and variety of its institutions, practitioners, and publications. As such, its ideals and services, whether formal or informal, continued to be important aspects of the overall medical or health strategies of individual Americans, at least those with sufficient means, irrespective of how much they utilized the mainline curative medical services.

The maintenance of a basic level of hygiene became an increasingly economic and class-related matter in late-nineteenth-century America, particularly in large cities. In fact, its pursuit was almost impossibly difficult for those who had to live in substandard urban tenements, accommodations for which neither landlords nor municipalities made much effort to dispose of the various human wastes. The slow extension of municipal water, sewer, and garbage-disposal systems in these areas, as well as the equally slow provision of plumbing, heating, and ventilation in the tenements, represented a chronic social disgrace, only sporadically alleviated by the activities of relevant reform movements.

The ultimate spreading of the municipal services did, of course, serve as an important stimulus to improved hygiene and cleanliness among all urban classes. But it was the upper and middle classes that were best able to take advantage of such developments. The coming of running water, in particular, not only made waste disposal safe and easy but made washing both easy and enjoyable for families with well-equipped bathrooms. By World War I a majority of city dwellers had probably attained such a standard. The development of electric fans, meanwhile, finally made it possible to more effectively circulate the air in urban apartments. At the same time, there was considerable continuing attention, among the educated and at least fairly well-off classes, to the care of their hygiene needs outside the home—walking, exercising, and obtaining other recreation.

The wealthy were able to pursue such activities at their athletic clubs, private pools, tennis courts, and bowling alleys. They had vacation homes at the beaches or in the mountains and also made visits to luxurious resort hotels. For various reasons, America's well-to-do steadily abandoned most of this country's great spas during this period, except where there were attractive golf courses or other social facilities to hold them. However, their belief in the curative powers of medicinal springs seems to have remained unshaken. By 1900, curative trips to the famous spas of Europe had substantially replaced their former trips of this nature to spas or water-cure hotels in the United States. And, thirty years later, in the single year of 1930 alone, some 100,000 Americans were reported to have taken treatments in these European institutions with their competent medical staffs and excellent facilities.

By the late-nineteenth century, higher incomes and improved transportation also enabled larger numbers of middle-class Americans to live well and healthfully and sometimes take vacations at resort hotels or private camps. Even the lower middle classes of the cities began to find better recreation facilities outside of their homes, albeit that these opportunities sometimes had moralistic strings attached to them. Conspicuous among these were the opportunities provided by the rapid post–Civil War expansion of the Young Men's Christian Association, the Young Men's Hebrew Association, and their counterparts for women. Most of the "Y's" introduced extensive hygiene and sports programs along with physical education facilities. Early in the twentieth century, moreover, the Boy Scout movement and other similar groups (some of them for girls) also began including recreational activities as parts of their character-building programs. Summer outdoor camps became prominent features of such activities among most of these groups.

Before the Civil War, philanthropists in the larger cities began sending selected "deserving" poor people, particularly children, if they met the moral specifications, out of the cities to summer camps. Considerably more comprehensive year-round programs and facilities for the poor, however, began to come into being during the 1880s and 1890s with the organization of urban settlement houses. Mostly these were church-supported and run by such well-educated women as Lillian Wald and Jane Addams. The settlements aimed primarily at the elevation and Americanization of immigrants. And, as integral parts of this, they provided various health-related services ranging from playgrounds and camps to free clinics, classes in hygiene and child care, and the help of visiting nurses. Nearly every large city relied heavily on its settlement houses during this period; there were over 450 of them by 1930. They did not pretend to meet all of the health-related needs of the slum dwellers, but as part of what their leaders regarded as their underlying "civilizing" mission, they performed important roles in teaching health practices, at least until the formation of appropriate public agencies.

Central among the exercise and recreation facilities at many of these and other social organizations were the gymnasiums. In fact, after a slow start in the early nineteenth century, the building of gymnasiums accelerated, late in the century, at a rate comparable to that of the building of hospitals. Before the Civil War most such establishments in the United States—probably not more than seventy in 1860—were those of the turnvereine, or gymnastic societies established by German immigrants. In addition, Dio Lewis, Catharine Beecher, and other hygienists, including several physicians, made some progress around mid-century at popularizing the virtues of calisthenics and formal exercises; the pursuit of such activities became known in some circles as "muscular Christianity." However, a substantial breakthrough in these pursuits did not come about until after the organization of early training programs in physical education in the late 1880s. From that point, within the next two decades alone, physical education programs were launched not only in some 500 YMCAs but in several hundred colleges, around 300 urban school systems, and numerous other clubs and institutions. This movement continued unabated across the country during the early twentieth century, gaining impetus from such sources as Theodore Roosevelt's advocacy of the strenuous life, eugenicists' worries about the deterioration of the white race, and the rise of such commercially successful body builders as Bernarr Macfadden. In the wake of these enthusiasms, innumerable new well-equipped gymnasiums rose around the country as conspicuous symbols of society's mixed dedication to exercise and better health.

Vying with the expanded facilities for exercise, physical education, and recreation as paths to better health in the United States was a rejuvenated gospel of healthful eating. Despite the campaigns of earlier health reformers, gastrointestinal problems caused by poorly prepared foods, unbalanced diets, atrociously fast eating, and gross overeating continued in disproportionate amounts among post–Civil War middle-class and upper-class populations. The seemingly infinite bounty produced by the country's agriculture was clearly one factor that contributed to overeating. At the same time, however, improved canning and food preservation technology, along with more rapid transportation of fresh fruits, vegetables, and dairy products, began to bring better balanced and nutritious meals increasingly within reach.

To promote better eating and nutrition became a central aim of a new generation of health educators and reformers of various kinds. In the process, Grahamism and some of the other older dietary regimens faded out of use or reappeared in different forms. Prominent among the turn-of-the-century reformers was Horace Fletcher who, in calling, among other things, for the prolonged chewing of food, attracted numerous followers for a time. Vegetarianism had a considerable resurgence as a key element in Fletcherism as well as in other regimens, notably those followed by the Seventh Day Adventists and other church groups. It was particularly prominent at the popular Battle Creek Sanitarium. There it was part of a comprehensive regimen of patient hygiene that was developed by John H. Kellogg. In his Battle Creek laboratory Kellogg also devised a number of food products, including the flaked cereal. But it was his brother W. K. Kellogg, along with C. W. Post, who went on to make these products the cornerstones of immensely profitable lines of prepared breakfast foods.

New impetus to more healthful eating also came, late in the nineteenth century, from laboratory science. During the 1890s, researches of the agricultural chemist Wilbur Atwater resulted, among other things, in the publication and distribution of the earliest tables giving caloric values for foods. Shortly after that, Russell Chittenden and his colleagues at Yale began conducting physiological and chemical studies on the effects of various diets on health. Researches of another agricultural chemist, Elmer McCollum, led to his discovery of vitamin A in 1913 and vitamin D in 1922. And, during the same decades, Joseph Goldberger headed a large Public Health Service study which firmly established pellagra as a food deficiency disease.

These and other scientific findings gradually had their effects on Americans' diets. The pasteurization of milk, first tried in this country in the 1890s, was extensively tested and debated before the process finally began to gain widespread acceptance and use during the World War I period. Atwater's caloric tables were widely distributed and utilized by hygienists, physicians, educators, and a new breed of professional nutritionists in schools, hospitals, and other institutions. Particularly influential in shaping this latter field was the Massachusetts Institute of Technology chemist Ellen Swallow Richards, whose New England Kitchen, which opened in Boston in 1890, provided good quality food to the poor. This philanthropy was subsequently duplicated in other cities. Richards, however, went on to make scientific nutrition a central part of the home economics movement, one which spread through colleges and schools across the nation soon after World War I.

Along with the flagrant dietary excesses, another major concern of hygienists and ordinary citizens alike was the continuing blight of excessive drinking of alcoholic beverages among individuals in all classes. Most of the concerned segments of society continued through this period to view alcoholism primarily as a moral and social problem. But hygienists, together with some physicians and scientists, persisted in regarding it also as a medical condition. Among the latter, neurologists and asylum physicians began giving increased attention to various physiological, psychological, and behavioral factors in alcoholism, while Raymond Pearl and others studied statistical and genetic aspects.

Around the turn of the century, orthodox medical groups and health officers played less conspicuous roles in the temperance movement than they had before the Civil War. However, not a few individual physicians continued to give the movement considerable priority. Such physicians and health reformers cooperated at various levels with the temperance societies. And many were key supporters of the political movement that resulted in passage of the Eighteenth

Amendment to the Constitution. The American Medical Association itself took a strong anti-alcohol position in 1917. However, by the mid-1920s it had reversed this stand following strong protests from the orthodox rank and file who considered alcohol an essential medicine.

Still another health-related issue, the birth control movement, owed even less than temperance did to physician support in its development during this period. During the mid-nineteenth-century decades there had been a fair amount of interest in birth control in American working-class families and feminist circles, from the viewpoint both of protecting womens' health and raising families' economic well-being. However, by the 1870s that movement had been largely suppressed by church and nativist groups who, for various reasons, wanted people to have more, not fewer, children. The regular medical profession contributed to this sentiment through its strong support for the federal and state "Comstock" laws of the 1870s. These laws classified contraceptive information and devices as immoral "obscenities" because they allegedly encouraged nonprocreative sexual activity. The effect was to drive the birth control movement underground for most of the next half-century. Most regular physicians, enthusiastically following the prevailing morality, declined through this period even to provide medical advice on the subject. The few doctors who were seriously interested in it were subjected to censorship and other difficulties when they wrote on scientific aspects of contraception.

Hygienists, teachers, and irregular physicians who attempted to continue their advocacy of birth control during this period were threatened with imprisonment and reduced to providing only an innocuous variety of sex education. In fact, few significant challenges to the restrictive laws were mounted before those made by Margaret Sanger during the World War I period. A nurse and radical reformer, Sanger began by being prosecuted for distributing birth control information, and in 1916 she was imprisoned when she opened a birth control clinic in Brooklyn. Thanks to broad judicial interpretations in this and other cases at the time, however, such activities gradually became feasible, particularly where physicians could be persuaded to participate. Sanger's subsequent role in the movement included her conduct of the *Birth Control Review* and her stimulation of a nationwide network of private birth control clinics for poor families. She also was the force behind various national committees and societies, some of which ultimately combined as the Planned Parenthood Federation of America. By World War II these bodies had done much both to make birth control widely available and to begin to make it respectable among the middle classes, even though the Comstock Act's restrictions were not formally repealed until 1971.

The birth control movement received surprising backing and encouragement after World War I from the Rockefellers and other American philanthropists. Some of this support went to assist the new clinics, to fund the preparation and distribution of authoritative sex education literature, and to back lobbying among members of the medical profession. The American Medical Association was finally persuaded to recognize contraception as a legitimate medical service in 1937. Meanwhile, beginning in the 1920s, foundation grants began supporting substantial research on sex-related matters. This ranged from studies on sexual psychology, endocrinology, and fertility to the development of cheaper and more effective contraceptives. Most researches were not very far advanced by the outbreak of World War II. Nevertheless, the birth control movement's efforts, among other things, had already served to highlight some of the broader health and medical needs of a great many Americans.

Society, Government, and the Expansion of Public Health

As in earlier periods, the activities of America's alternative health movements, along with those of the medical establishment, focused essentially on the individual. But there remained ever larger matters affecting the health of people and communities in the aggregate, matters that were outside the scope both of regular and irregular medical groups and certainly beyond the capacity of most individuals to do anything about. Above all, the actual and threatened spread of infectious diseases among large numbers of people in the deteriorating post–Civil War urban centers required very large measures. To cope with such problems, despite the prevalent laissez-faire attitudes of the day, members of post–Civil War and early-twentieth-century society turned increasingly to governments for help. Following a gradual coming together of political, medical, and social reform energies and pressures, the circumstances were finally created for a proliferation at all levels of government of agencies with public health responsibilities. Working in a framework of changing medical and scientific concepts, the various agencies and departments steadily extended the reach of public health work to new or neglected segments of society. As they did so, they began to give new hygienic attention to America's habitats and to upgrade them in important ways.

This postwar efflorescence of public health activity, like its more limited earlier manifestations, took place at first mainly in the large cities. To be sure, such activity, like other new urban governmental operations, had to overcome a heavy incubus of political pressure and inertia. "Progress" often seemed to come about only with the periodic threat of epidemics or the launching of reform movements after especially flagrant sanitary scandals. However, with the rapid increases of population and of industry, the late-nineteenth-century accumulations of wastes built up so much more rapidly than previously as to make expeditious action to deal with them seem essential to the survival of the cities.

Certain post–Civil War reformers and entrepreneurs drew attention to the role of individual households in this process. And some capitalized on it commercially by actively promoting better home sanitation for the upper classes, specifically through popularizing and marketing improved plumbing devices such as drains, sinks, cesspools, and above all, toilets. One of these popularizers, George E. Waring, was said to have shocked some of his readers in the *Atlantic Monthly* and *Scribners* by the "infinite gusto" with which he portrayed the health dangers from sewer gas presumed to be spread by faulty plumbing. Significant sanitary improvement did result from such warnings, at least in the homes of the well-to-do. However, Waring and his contemporaries soon realized that broader successes along these lines could not be expected until the development of community sewerage systems, water works, and other sanitary facilities was much further along. Several of these individuals thus also began to apply their sanitary expertise to the larger public projects.

During the immediate postwar period, several American cities resumed work on sanitary projects that had been interrupted by the war. Numerous others began to launch more modern sewerage and water supply systems based on recent European and British models. By the 1880s and 1890s, a major sanitary upsurge, centered generally in departments of public works, was under way and spreading rapidly in the American cities. Crucial to this development was the emergence of this country's first generation of professional sanitary engineers, conspicuous among them such men as Waring, Rudolph Hering, and Samuel Gray. As consultants, these competent and often authoritarian individuals designed new sanitary systems for hundreds of Gilded Age cities and towns. Some of them also experimented with modes of garbage disposal, organized and ran street cleaning departments, continued to devise home plumbing fixtures, laid out public parks, and continued to serve as publicists for sanitary works.

Because of the constant expansion of urban populations, many of the larger sanitary works were never really completed. Moreover, their construction often served to compound the public health problems of cities, particularly when, as so often occurred, the effluents of sewer systems along with the collections of garbage and trash were simply deposited into the nearest body of water. By the 1920s and 1930s, virtually every major American river, lake, and harbor was heavily polluted from such effluents, together with those given off by industry. And the provision of adequate water purification, sewage treatment, and garbage disposal plants proved to be about as slow and costly as the building of the aqueducts and sewers themselves.

In important respects, however, the various engineering works substantially offset rather than added to the pollution produced by the industrial establishments of the period. Through water, sewerage, and garbage disposal systems, city inhabitants now received a demonstrably large measure of protection from the diseases that were often transmitted in human excreta. Most human wastes could now be removed from the cities on a systematic basis. As such, the sanitary facilities quickly became indispensable to modern city life. Whatever their shortcomings, they altered the physical environment of the early-twentieth-century American city sufficiently to make it a substantially more pleasant and healthful place to live in than it had been fifty years earlier.

Playing more modest roles in the cities' hygienic build-up for some time were the physician health officers, sanitary inspectors, and other employees of the health departments. Given the prevailing ethos of the period, these individuals, like other municipal employees, were generally at the mercy of constantly shifting political fortunes, and their work suffered accordingly. Nevertheless, they were made responsible for a considerable variety of activities. Health departments of the period often provided free vaccination against smallpox to immigrants, schoolchildren, and others. And eventually, in the effort to prevent the spread of this and other infectious diseases, their employees frequently quarantined the sick, placarded residences, and, using elaborate equipment, disinfected the interiors of the latter.

However, reflecting the immediate postbellum period's predominantly environmental or anticontagionist outlook on health and disease, most of the health officers' time, and that of their staffs, was for some time taken up with detailed sanitary concerns and chores: eradicating "filth" in the immediate environment. Especially prominent among these activities was the investigation and removal of public "nuisances" that were associated with ill health and disease—

conditions such as decaying garbage, leaking or foul-smelling privies, dead animals or trash in vacant lots and streets. They likewise inspected food in the markets, checked ventilation and waste disposal in tenements, and were sometimes responsible for garbage collection and disposal. As the nineteenth century went on, the health officers frequently had to prod the city government to speed up sewer construction and then to sue landlords to connect their tenements to the sewer systems. In many cities the health officer was also designated as registrar of vital statistics. To the extent that the data were complete, his analyses of the distribution of deaths from various causes could tell much about the sanitary state of the respective wards and precincts.

From around the mid-1880s the city health departments began to undergo profound changes in the light of the new knowledge and methods of the bacteriological age. Central in these was the onset of a fundamental questioning of much of the departments' routine environmental cleansing activity. Gradually assuming direction of a few of the country's health departments was a new generation of physician health officers who were convinced that specific germs or other microscopic organisms rather than miasmas or general filthy conditions were responsible for the spread of most urban "crowd" diseases. And they began to modify traditional activities accordingly.

By soon after 1900, with privy vaults disappearing and other urgent environmental problems coming under control in some cities, the new-style health officers began to give less emphasis to garbage collection, nuisance removal, and other traditional work of sanitary police. The ideal, only slowly realized, was to transfer such activities to other municipal departments. In their place, they steadily introduced highly specific measures aimed at identifying particular organisms of given diseases and preventing their spread. As worked out by Charles V. Chapin in Providence, Hermann Biggs in New York, George Goler in Rochester, and other turn-of-the-century city and state health officers, such measures evolved by World War I into a scientific and highly systematic approach known as the "New Public Health." Although under this the building of basic sanitary facilities was granted to be essential in every community, once they were completed members of the new generation of health officers did their best to give up activities that did not affect given diseases directly.

A crucial first step leading to the New Public Health was the establishment and spread of public health laboratories. These were originally used primarily for testing the purity of public water supplies and the effectiveness of filtration systems. By the mid-1890s, however, following the initiative of the New York City Health Department, the laboratories also began to make routine diagnostic tests to verify suspected cases of diphtheria, typhoid fever, tuberculosis, scarlet fever, and other common infectious diseases of cities. In addition, at about the same time, the laboratories of a few large city health departments initiated the manufacture and distribution of sera and vaccines, notably diphtheria antitoxin. They quickly withdrew from such enterprises, however, as the pharmaceutical industry became more heavily involved in them.

As the laboratory diagnosis of disease improved, city health officers extended their efforts to obtain ordinances requiring physicians to report cases of infectious disease. And, as man's knowledge of the behavior of bacteria and other organisms increased, the health officers refined and changed their measures to control such diseases. They replaced many of their nuisance inspectors with medical inspectors. They began to give up the elaborate apparatus they had used for disinfecting household objects. And they devoted increased attention to the sources of the continued high mortality rates among infants and children. Much of this latter effort concentrated on the promotion of breast-feeding, but also on improving the public milk supply through such steps as the creation of milk stations, inspection of dairies, and eventually the use of pasteurization.

The new health officers also greatly expanded their departments' health education programs. One key step was to engage visiting nurses to carry the precepts of personal cleanliness and hygiene to school children and immigrant families. Equally important was the dissemination of up-to-date information to the general public, through lectures and newspapers, on recent medical discoveries and on the various modes of disease transmission. And sometimes a resort to personal example seemed to be useful. At the Providence City Hall, health officer Charles V. Chapin for some time went to the lengths of conspicuously wiping doorknobs on entering and leaving the public restrooms in order to show the need for individuals to protect themselves against germs, though the act resulted in considerable snickering behind his back.

Some cities also experimented with new types of infectious disease hospitals; the pioneering institutions in the United States were in Providence and New York City. These hospitals proved to be far cries from the infamous pesthouses that had stood menacingly near cities' limits since time immemorial, though it took some time for public opinion to accept them. In the modern versions, it was argued that neither hospitals nor patients were threats to the rest of the community so long as cross-infection was properly guarded against. This was ensured by enforcing strict aseptic methods, or cleanliness, on the part of the nurses and physicians. At first, such hospitals tended to admit only individuals suffering from common infectious diseases that were not alarming or in social disrepute. However, as the twentieth century went on, even cases of tuberculosis, venereal diseases, and other infections were admitted.

Many of the post–Civil War changes in city public health work were stimulated and facilitated by a slow but steady professionalization of the field, a process that included the usual formation of specialty societies as well as a variety of periodicals and texts. These institutions and tools were shaped to meet the diverse needs of the sanitary engineers, visiting nurses, statisticians, and other professionals as well as the physician health officers. Similarly, academic courses on various aspects of sanitation, bacteriology, and public health were introduced during the 1880s and 1890s. And these expanded into separate departments and schools of public health at several of the larger universities during the next few decades.

Still another major aspect of public health change was the emergence of state departments, and boards, of health. This development proved to be the key step in the initiation of significant hygienic organizations and services in a large proportion of the counties, towns, and other small communities around the country.

Formation of the Massachusetts State Board of Health in 1869 provided the model for numerous subsequent state boards; it was followed closely by the establishment of boards in some fifteen other states during the 1870s, and in many of the remaining states during the next two decades. The early state boards were normally limited in their powers to giving advice, carrying out investigations within very limited budgets, sometimes running state vital statistics registration systems, and generally encouraging the organization of permanent local health boards and sanitary services. But gradually they were given additional authority: to require sanitary reports from local communities; to establish statewide health standards or procedures; sometimes to enforce state laws; and generally to extend health services and health education efforts where there had not been any.

As centers of hygienic activity, the state boards gradually took on a variety of experts. These individuals became involved in numerous activities, many of which were beyond the scope of most local health departments: the inspection and supervision of food, water, and milk supplies; the planning of large sewerage and water supply systems; the investigation and enforcement of occupational health and safety; the licensure of such professions as physicians, undertakers, and barbers; and the statewide dissemination of health information. Some state boards had quarantine responsibilities. Most eventually began to provide laboratory diagnostic services to physicians and local health officials. Others undertook significant research functions: the design and testing of water and sewerage purification techniques; the improvement of ventilation; the statistical analysis of disease and death data. And all became involved in epidemiological studies and the tracing of disease outbreaks.

Within states, the extension of public health agencies and services to poor or rural areas was notoriously slow. Similarly, from state to state, the pace of creating and developing state health institutions was consistently determined by such factors as levels of population density, urban development, industrialization, and wealth. The 1914 A.M.A. survey of state boards of health conducted by Charles V. Chapin confirmed that at that time the best state boards were mostly in the Northeast and North-Central regions. State health departments and programs in the South had recently been noticeably strengthened, mainly through assistance provided by the Rockefeller Sanitary Commission. However, few public health institutions or services of any kind were yet provided in most of the predominantly rural, poorly developed, and sparsely settled western states. The states' capacities even to obtain accurate and full records of deaths within their borders followed this same pattern. Most northern and eastern states were maintaining such data systematically before 1900. But nearly a dozen western states still lacked the needed mechanisms for this in the early 1920s.

The federal government became progressively more involved in this particular public health problem from the 1880s, with new efforts on the part of United States Census officials to encourage and aid the states in improving their birth and death statistics. To be sure, this was an extremely modest commitment, for any attempt to give the government a larger role in health matters was still subjected to all the same obstacles that the states and cities encountered from Gilded Age politics and laissez-faire economics. Post–Civil War society was increasingly aware, however, that cholera, yellow fever, and other epidemic disease threats not only frequently transcended state borders but were beyond the capacities of most states to cope with. Many came to believe it incumbent upon the federal government to assume greater authority in such matters at an early date.

Reflecting this sentiment, national medical and public health societies throughout the 1870s pushed actively for legislation to create a federal health agency. The National Board of Health, established in 1879 and dominated by such individuals as the Army's John Shaw Billings, James L. Cabell of Virginia, and Stephen Smith of New York City, existed briefly as an important step in this direction. But Congress withdrew support for it after only a few years when its work stirred up states rights opposition and Washington political antagonisms. As a result, throughout the rest of the nineteenth century and beyond, the federal health-related activities that were undertaken continued to consist of bits and pieces of programs located in various governmental departments.

The Army Medical Department, during this period, continued to extend its national medical and public health activities. Increasingly conspicuous was the Department's growing involvement in research and its striking contributions to preventive medicine. George Sternberg was foremost among the medical officers who, during the 1880s and 1890s, began to bring the knowledge and methods of the bacteriological age into army medicine. This was not only due to his original research and authorship of America's first text in the field but to his creation in 1893 of the Army Medical School. Largely through this institution, by the outbreak of the Spanish-American War a substantial number of the Army's medical officers had received training in modern medical science and preventive medicine. The school also provided essential laboratory backup services for wartime and postwar medical activities.

Walter Reed, an instructor at the School and curator at the Army Medical Museum, gained scientific attention for his role in the notable Reed-Vaughan-Shakespeare survey of epidemic typhoid fever in United States military camps during the Spanish-American War. Among other things, the authors demonstrated the importance of "well carriers" in transmitting this disease. Reed then went on, with the other members of a special Army inquiry board, to gain still wider acclaim for their definitive studies in postwar Cuba on the etiology and transmission of yellow fever.

Another Army medical officer, William C. Gorgas, became almost equally noted during the Army's follow-up of the yellow fever board's demonstrations. Concentrating on eradication of the *Aedes aegypti* mosquito, Gorgas put into effect sanitary measures which in 1900 effectively rid Havana of yellow fever. Later on, between 1904 and 1905, he also supervised measures that essentially eliminated both yellow fever and malaria from the Panama Canal Zone. Subsequently, other Army medical officers, along with Public Health Service physicians, continued sanitary work and studies of tropical diseases abroad, though particularly in Puerto Rico, the Philippines, and other corners of America's new colonial empire. In fact, in various locations Army personnel continued to play innovative roles in research and preventive medicine, not least of which was the making of vaccination against typhoid a standard procedure among United States troops.

Seeking to play a somewhat comparable public health role among America's civilian population during this same period was the Marine Hospital Service. This agency was formed within the Treasury Department in 1870 to administer the government's scattered marine hospitals. By the 1890s it was also assigned maritime quarantine responsibilities. It quickly gained favorable public and congressional attention in this work, particularly with its vigorous and largely successful efforts to prevent the entry of cholera and bubonic plague into American ports. Around 1900, moreover, the Service began to broaden its activities within the country, particularly those relating to the communicable diseases. Prominent among these steps was the steady enlargement of its Hygienic Laboratory, and through it, the extension of diagnostic services to the marine hospitals and to state health departments. The Laboratory also acquired authority to establish nationwide standards for and regulate the use of sera and other biological products.

During the first quarter of the century, among other projects, the Service launched an important series of field investigations of diseases. While these activities served all geographical areas of the country, the Service's scientists gained particular prominence for work done in those states or regions with poorly developed local health departments and services. These included, for example, investigations by Charles Wardell Stiles of hookworm disease among southern poor whites, surveys by Leslie Lumsden of the incidence of typhoid fever, studies by George McCoy and Edward Francis of tularemia in the West, and the program of Joseph Goldberger that established the relationship of diet deficiency to the incidence of pellagra in the South. In the aggregate, along with campaigns against trachoma among Indian groups, studies of Rocky Mountain spotted fever, and other projects, these Public Health Service activities constituted the nation's first extended program to deal with serious illness in its rural and remote habitats.

Many of these activities included systematic efforts to improve the basic sanitary habits of rural populations. Of them, none was more important than the labors of Lumsden and Stiles in designing, popularizing, and educating people to use their insect-proof sanitary privy. As a result of that work, Stiles, with his heavily Prussian bearing, gained the nickname around Washington as the Service's "*Privy Counsellor.*"

Impressive as it was in such ways, the Service's pre–World War

I growth did not begin to satisfy the hopes and expectations of numerous reformers, officials, health professionals, and educators. Responding to these dissatisfactions, a Committee of One Hundred on National Health was formed under Yale's Irving Fisher to represent such individuals in seeking, among other things, a more aggressive federal role in public health. Between 1906 and 1910 this Committee worked for legislation that would bring together the Marine Hospital Service and the government's other health-related programs, including those for Indians, federal prisoners, and miners, in a single cabinet level department of health and to give it substantial added areas of authority. While this movement ultimately failed, due partly to powerful antimonopolistic and antimedical establishment sentiment, the Marine Hospital Service in 1912 was at least given a new name, the Public Health Service, one that suggested a potentially broader mission for the future. Still, for several more decades, major nonmilitary health programs of the federal government continued to be dispersed among several agencies.

The Department of Agriculture had begun taking on several such activities in the 1880s. Its Bureau of Chemistry under Harvey Wiley early became involved in the analysis of food adulterants and preservatives from the viewpoint both of nutrition and safety. The Bureau of Animal Industry, in turn, conducted extensive pathological researches, most prominent of which were Daniel Salmon's work on hog cholera and Theobald Smith's pathbreaking study of Texas cattle fever. The Bureau in the 1890s also began inspecting meat products intended for the export market.

The programs of both bureaus were noticeably expanded soon after 1900 as a result of powerful pressures from consumer and medical groups, together with exposés by several of the decade's muckraking writers. Particularly influential were Samuel Hopkins Adams's articles in *Collier's* magazine on the country's patent medicine evils and Upton Sinclair's novel *The Jungle*, which presented a revolting picture of conditions in turn-of-the-century meat-packing establishments. Congress responded to these pressures by enacting both a new and broader meat inspection bill and the first federal food and drug act, administration of which was assigned to the Department of Agriculture. While generally beneficial in their effects, the provisions of the Food and Drug Act turned out to be vulnerable to manufacturers' evasions and pressures during the subsequent decades. As such they were considerably weakened and were only restored and strengthened in 1938, with passage of a comprehensive new act to regulate foods, drugs, and cosmetics.

Another federal health agency, one with more modest beginnings in this period, was the Children's Bureau. The Bureau was one of several private and public agencies created by turn-of-the-century pediatricians, health officials, social workers, legislators, and others in an attempt to reduce the appalling infant mortality from diarrheas and other diseases. S. Josephine Baker set the pattern for governmental action with her pioneering child hygiene program within the New York City Department of Health in 1907. Other city and state health departments followed within a few years, while Congress created the Children's Bureau in 1912 as a part of the Department of Labor. Among its early activities, the Bureau attempted to improve birth and death statistics, surveyed current child health activities already in progress, and began significant programs of research and education in child nutrition, maternal health, mental health, and related matters. After 1916 it took over enforcement of the first federal child labor law, and in 1921 it also became responsible for administering the Sheppard-Towner Act. This Act created a program of grants to assist states in developing activities to combat infant and maternal mortality. Before being terminated by Congress in 1929 the program resulted in the creation of some 3,000 child health and prenatal centers throughout the country.

Playing major roles in the late nineteenth and early twentieth century, both in stimulating the creation of official health agencies at all levels of government and then in supplementing their services, were several types of new private enterprises. Most conspicuous of these was a burgeoning array of local, state, and national voluntary health organizations. Volunteerism on behalf of the country's public health had, to be sure, such distinguished earlier precedents as the various Civil War sanitary commissions and, since the 1880s, the American Red Cross. This latter body, in addition to the war and disaster relief activities launched by its forceful founder, Clara Barton, eventually went on to initiate important programs in such areas as water safety, first aid, public health nursing, and health education.

Many of the newer voluntary health bodies organized first at local levels but rapidly expanded to include state and national organizations. Most were composed variously of health professionals, academics, and highly dedicated laymen and women—civic leaders, reformers, philanthropists, and others. Impatient with the slow extension of governmental health work, such individuals took it upon themselves to raise large amounts of money, conduct surveys, stimulate research, distribute health education materials, and undertake other measures, often pertaining to specific diseases.

Setting the pattern for these organizations at the national level was the National Association for the Study and Prevention of Tuberculosis. Established in 1904, this organization, together with its local counterparts and official health departments, achieved great success during the next several decades in obtaining the reporting of tuberculosis cases, stimulating the establishment of tuberculosis sanatoria, and promoting the improvement of personal hygienic habits among the public. Despite their extensive general importance for public health, the role of such steps in the contemporaneous decline of tuberculosis was undoubtedly less than that of America's steady rise in living standards. Nevertheless, by the 1920s health officers were noticeably heartened by the results of the antituberculosis campaign. One side effect was their discovery that spitting was "becoming a lost art."

The national tuberculosis association was followed rapidly by bodies devoted to child health (1909), mental hygiene (1909), public health nursing (1912), cancer control (1913), and other concerns. The enthusiasms and energies of these organizations were of immense value in extending the reach of local public health efforts. However, the agencies frequently overlapped in scope and became increasingly competitive in their money-raising campaigns. Efforts to organize joint appeals or otherwise coordinate the various campaigns began in some communities during the 1920s and 1930s. But the freewheeling nature of these philanthropies changed little up into the 1980s.

An additional supplement to early-twentieth-century public health services came from activities of a few large life insurance companies. Such firms had long understood that keeping the aggregate members of society alive longer could lead to greater corporate profits, and this philosophy now fit in well with the various ideological contradictions of the Progressive Era. Some companies, through their actuaries, had been lending their support to the improvement of public sanitary works and vital statistics since the mid-nineteenth century. Now their activities broadened. The Life Extension Institute, on behalf of the industry, before 1914 began offering free medical examinations around the country. In another direction, Frederick L. Hoffmann of the Prudential Insurance Company organized and carried out important quantitative studies on such topics as the diseases and mortality of southern blacks, the distribution of cancer, and the incidence of tuberculosis in the "dusty trades." Even more far-reaching, under the leadership of Lee K. Frankel and Louis I. Dublin, were the programs of the Metropolitan Life Insurance Company, particularly its financial support of health-related organizations and local health departments, its encouragement of public health nursing, and its development and distribution of health education materials. At the same time, however, the vigorous opposition of the life insurance companies did a great deal, between 1910 and 1920, to bring about the defeat of the early attempts to obtain legislation for an American system of national health insurance.

A third type of private enterprise that began to have important health-related objectives during this period, and with somewhat more complex motivations than the insurance companies, was the new philanthropic foundation. From their beginnings, many of these organizations were heavily interested in medical education and the medical sciences. But a considerable number concentrated their resources largely on public health matters. The Milbank Memorial Fund began such support in 1905. After 1907, the Russell Sage Foundation, among other programs, organized sanitary surveys in several cities and conducted specialized health demonstrations in others. Meanwhile, these and numerous other early foundations also funded laboratories and research projects that had great public health significance, particularly the investigation of infectious diseases and the development of sera or vaccines.

Among the various foundations, none matched the Rockefeller philanthropies in resources or in the scope of their public health programs. The Rockefeller Sanitary Commission's 1909–1914 campaign against hookworm disease in the South, in fact, represented a larger investment in a specific public health problem than even the federal government was as yet willing to make. While that campaign did not by any means fully eradicate the disease, it did prove to be immensely important in strengthening southern state health departments, stimulating the building of rural sanitary facilities, and providing basic health education to a large population. The Sanitary Commission also led directly to the organization of the extensive international health programs of the Rockefeller Foundation. One phase of the Foundation's activities, the training of foreign health personnel, led in turn to a major commitment on its part to high quality public health education. In the United States this included large financial support for new or reorganized public health schools at Johns Hopkins (1917), Harvard (1922), and several other universities. These schools reflected better than almost any other element the continuing steady transformation of public health work into an ever more specialized scientific profession.

For all of its new scientific proficiency and hosts of public and private agencies, public health, and with it the ideal of preventive medicine, failed to take hold in the United States to the extent that its adherents had expected. Baltimore's liberal physician and historian Henry E. Sigerist in the 1930s attributed this to some extent to America's individualistic social and economic traditions but primarily to the indifference or opposition of a conservative medical establishment. With the increasing medicalization of public health work at this time, physicians were in great demand as health officers and administrators. But medical students continued overwhelmingly to opt instead for better paying careers in private practice. The American Medical Association, in turn, not only dropped much of its earlier support of sanitation and public health, but by the 1920s had adopted policies that were actively hostile to preventive and public medicine. Prominent among these stands, it strongly opposed compulsory health insurance, fought against the Sheppard-Towner Act, and originally resisted proposals for both group medical care and prepaid medical care as being "socialistic" in nature.

America's involvement in World War I required the government to utilize both curative and preventive medicine to the full. The massive temporary military medical establishment that sprang up almost overnight in 1917 did employ, in fact, not only the entire range of new knowledge, therapies, methods, and instruments, but the various kinds of institutions that had recently evolved in every field of medicine and medical science. The very variety of health professionals that were mustered for the war effort reflected the new character and complexity of twentieth-century medicine. There were not only surgeons, nurses, pharmacists, orderlies, and ambulance drivers as in previous wars, but sanitary engineers, laboratory technicians, dentists, and specialists of every stripe—psychiatrists, neurologists, epidemiologists, dermatologists, nutritionists, ophthalmologists, immunologists, and many more. And testimony of their collective value came after the war when the statistical record revealed that, for the first time in this country's history, there had been fewer deaths from diseases than from battle wounds.

The accomplishment of this record was achieved by innovation in many areas of World War I medicine. Among these, the physical examination of recruits, more thorough than ever before and including IQ tests, weeded out startling numbers of young men with some disqualifying physical or mental condition. In another major step, the sharply rising incidence of venereal disease among the troops led the nation to mount an unparalleled campaign of education and prophylaxis against the evil, in civilian communities as well as in the camps. At the front lines in Europe, dysentery and diarrheal diseases continued to be serious because of difficulties in enforcing sanitation and personal hygiene. Some of the other familiar camp diseases, however, by World War I were fairly well controlled, typhoid by vaccination and typhus by delousing. To some extent laboratories were established to provide diagnostic back-up.

Meanwhile, in the military hospitals, army surgeons undertook a far greater variety of operations than had their predecessors in earlier wars. Using asepsis, anesthetics, and other still newer techniques, they were now able to save many wounded who had serious internal and head injuries. At the same time, hospital personnel had to deal with the victims of a deadly new weapon, poison gas, along with shellshock on an unprecedented scale. Numerically, however, the worst disease condition of all came just after the end of the war with the onset of epidemic influenza. This was a worldwide pandemic that devastated not only the troops who were still in uniform but the civilian populations, and before which the leaders of scientific medicine and public health confessed themselves to be virtually helpless.

While America's toll of World War I dead and wounded did not approach that of the Civil War, nevertheless thousands of disabled soldiers required continuing hospitalization and rehabilitation after the coming of peace. In 1921 the government hospitals that were caring for such veterans were placed in a new Veterans Bureau, an agency that was enlarged in 1930 and renamed the Veterans Administration. Besides these post–World War I hospitals, the Administration took over the previously existing soldiers' homes, the management of disability compensation mechanisms, rehabilitation programs, and other medical programs for the veterans.

These federal provisions for veterans' care, along with those for maternal and child health, stood out as conspicuous exceptions in an overall pattern of official indifference to human needs which characterized the United States during the 1920s. The onset of this period of neglect was signaled in 1920 by the call of the future president, Warren Harding, for a "return to normalcy," an appeal that swept the Republicans into national office and in effect kept them there until 1933. For them, the return to normalcy meant making a sharp break with the social and political reform spirit of the Progressive movement. It stood above all for a cutback of government activities and expenditures, a virtual end to government interference with private enterprise, and increased support of commerce and industry by government. Socially, the politics of normalcy were supported or accompanied by a resurgence of nativism and intolerance on a massive scale. This was reflected variously by the enactment of major restrictions on immigration, widespread hostility toward labor unions and political extremists, and by the flourishing of antiblack, Catholic, and Jewish sentiment, not only in the Ku Klux Klan but throughout much of the rest of society.

Health and medicine were deeply affected by many of these developments. The campaign for governmental health insurance was sidetracked throughout the decade, while the Sheppard-Towner Act's programs were discontinued in 1929, within a few years of their beginning. The conservative policies of the American Medical Association and other segments of the medical establishment were greatly reinforced. Pharmaceutical manufacturers and other medical industries flourished in the probusiness atmosphere. Corporate and organizational ties as well as professional links became closer and more complex between many of the orthodox medical institutions and organizations—industries, societies, research institutes, medical schools, and foundations. Hospitals steadily took on more of the traits of businesses and, late in the pre–World War II period, began to experiment with new proposals for health care finance. Meanwhile, large numbers of government physicians, scientists, and officials of the 1920s, like the legislators, tended to acquiesce in the free enterprise outlook and objectives of the decade. This had the effect of bringing many of their agencies and regulatory bodies into a close community of interest and outlook with the various conservative institutions, interests, and leadership elements of the country's orthodox medical establishment, often to the detriment of other health care interests.

Under the "normalcy" and free enterprise of the 1920s, America's middle and upper classes commanded high levels of medical and health care. However, the same could not be said for the economically and socially disadvantaged. Large numbers of the nation's working-class people, blacks, recent immigrants, Indians, farmers, and others continued to have only the most minimal access to health care and sanitary services. As such, they were highly vulnerable healthwise to economic changes; in fact, for farmers and others such dislocations were beginning to have serious effects long before the end of the period. As early as 1923, for instance, the journalist Samuel Hopkins Adams reported that the country doctor was fast becoming a vanishing species, large numbers having already moved to the cities after World War I to become specialists. Farm families, he found, increasingly despaired of obtaining medical care for even their seriously ill infants.

By the 1930s, these and other segments of American society found themselves in still greater medical need as part of the accumulating distresses brought on by the Great Depression. Many of the urgent needs were highlighted in 1932 by national public health leaders as parts of an important Report on the Costs of Medical Care. Adopting parts of this report, the planners and pragmatists who went on to fashion the New Deal made medical and public health relief a significant if not central part of their economic relief and recovery agencies.

The Federal Emergency Relief Administration, for one, in addition to conducting an extensive "health inventory," supplied funds for rural health programs. The Farm Security Administration, through support for a system of medical cooperatives, provided group medical care for many of the poorest farmers, sharecroppers, migrant workers, and their families. Both the Works Progress Administration and the Public Works Administration, on the other hand, provided various health services as well as funds for new public sanitary works and hospitals, while the Civil Works Administration helped in the financing of disease control projects. Farthest reaching of all was the Social Security Act. Not only did this Act provide a source of income for the unemployed, but its grant funds brought about the restoration, beginning in 1937, of many of the Sheppard-Towner Act's programs in maternal and child health. Other funds helped materially, not only in reviving but in extending the activities of state and local health departments.

With these latter programs, the federal government's permanent role in medicine and health was once again significantly expanded. And, with the creation in 1939 of the Federal Security Agency, significant progress was finally achieved in the effort to bring the government's scattered civilian health-related responsibilities and agencies together under a common administration. By the time of America's entrance into World War II, the laissez-faire medical attitudes and approaches of the 1920s had once more been replaced by a multifaceted governmental commitment to participate with nongovernmental agencies in applying and distributing the benefits of modern science, medicine, and public health.

CHAPTER 4

AMERICA SINCE 1940:
PROSPEROUS MEDICINE AND
ELUSIVE HEALTH

A S THE DECADE of the 1940s began, American governments—federal, state, and local—were infinitely more involved in medical affairs than they had been during the 1870s and 1880s. At the same time, American citizens had gained a degree of confidence in physicians and other health professionals that would have been unimaginable to their great-grandparents. A large percentage of them utilized modern mainline medicine regularly and had come to appreciate its virtues and potential. Nevertheless, many continued to look outside the medical establishment for satisfaction of certain needs bearing on health and physical well-being. Nationwide, the New Deal had heightened peoples' perception that the various health and medical services were rights of citizens just as the franchise was, with the result that governments and society as a whole were now committed, at least in theory, to making them easier to obtain and more equitable for all classes of citizens.

The demands of World War II interrupted the implementation of these and other medical and social programs. They also interrupted or diverted the development of medical care institutions, medical industries, and medical research. However, the ultimate ending of the war permitted a rapid resumption of growth in all of these areas. With postwar growth, many of the modes, circumstances, and traditions of medical care, like other aspects of American life, underwent further radical alteration. Such changes, together with an unsettling erosion of the quality of life in Americans' habitats, stimulated a renewed popular questioning of mainline medical philosophy, some resistance to its techniques, and a new reaching out to alternative or supplemental roads to health. Nevertheless, by the 1970s and 1980s, the overall pursuit of medicine and health in its manifold forms—private and public, establishment and nonestablishment—had emerged as one of the nation's largest and most costly enterprises,

125

second in magnitude, in fact, only to the military. But conspicuous inequities persisted in peoples' access to the various health-related resources and services.

World War II and Its Medical Aftermath

World War II provided a new set of human and health concerns to cope with, problems that pushed the disabilities, social dislocations, and economic breakdowns of the Great Depression into the background. For the United States, mobilization and pursuit of the war involved the mustering, training, and support of over 12 million individuals in the fighting forces for more than five years, together with the concurrent redirection and exploitation of industry, labor, agriculture, science, and the economy on a huge scale. America ultimately emerged from the war with its industry and economy in full health once again. However, in the prosecution of the war it had suffered a loss of 325,000 killed and 700,000 wounded.

Medical organization for the war—the third in less than fifty years—was once again a vast enterprise in itself. Briefly summarized, it involved, as had every conflict, building and equipping hospitals and other facilities in camps or installations at home and abroad, staffing these institutions with the necessary medical professionals and technicians, and keeping them supplied. For this particular conflict, the process proved remarkably thorough and effective. In fact, the World War II military forces were able to virtually replicate and often even to exceed the health care facilities that the average American by then had become used to at home. Thanks to them, as well as to such new therapeutic aids as penicillin and the sulfa drugs, to improved treatment of trauma shock and uses of blood plasma, and to rapid new modes of evacuating the wounded, the proportion of fatalities among the wounded was far less than in World War I.

As the hostilities went on, the country's medical research community became increasingly involved in war-related problems. Particularly crucial was the intensive scientific effort that was undertaken to bring penicillin into large-scale production. The military action in Africa and the Pacific, moreover, stimulated intensive research on tropical diseases and the development of new drugs to use against them. Of the latter, the development of a quinine substitute became especially urgent when normal supplies of quinine were cut off during the fighting. Meanwhile, America's medical industries produced a vast continuous flow of instruments, prosthetics, bandages, and other medical supplies, not only for the American forces but for Allied troops in every theater of war.

The ending of World War II left the United States with a number of, by then, familiar human and medical obligations. The country now had a new generation of war dead to mourn. And it had a new population of war-wounded to care for and to attempt to rehabilitate. Government and society moved rapidly to provide the necessary hospital and other services for the wounded veterans. And by-and-large they seem to have done better in this than previous generations had. At the same time, Congress also proved sensitive to the needs of the unwounded veterans by providing for large-scale educational, counseling, and retraining programs for this group.

Apart from these domestic effects, World War II also had significant international medical consequences, among them an accelerated alteration of America's medical relations with much of the rest of the world. The ending of the war left large parts of the various European countries physically devastated, with economies exhausted and sometimes with essential facilities destroyed and services seriously disrupted. The situation in those countries was paralleled by the rapid postwar dissolution of Europe's colonial empires in Asia and Africa and by their transformation into independent but often poverty-stricken nations. Medical services and institutions were among the elements that badly needed postwar support or rehabilitation, both in these new countries and in Europe. Since the United States, almost alone among the great powers, emerged from the war in a state of full economic and military strength, it was uniquely able to provide such assistance. And it had political as well as humanitarian motives to do so.

The postwar decades thus witnessed a broad-based United States involvement in world medical recovery. Much of this consisted of direct assistance by the American government to the individual countries, but this was supplemented by important programs of foundations, the Red Cross, and other private groups. In Europe, American aid went for such objectives as the replacement of hospitals, the rebuilding of sanitary systems, and the resumption of medical research. And in the former colonies and Third World, funds were provided for at least a part of the immense needs for medical education, sanitary facilities, clinics, disease eradication programs, population control, improved nutrition, and other essentials. Substantial American assistance was also channeled through the World Health Organization and the health-related programs of other international bodies.

As a result of these various programs and initiatives, American orthodox medicine became the new model after which many other countries, particularly those that were receptive to Western ideas, fashioned their own modern medical institutions and services. The United States was now recognized as possessing a large proportion of the world's best equipped and most productive biomedical research centers and hospitals. It published more than its share of the scientific and medical specialty journals. Moreover, climaxing the reversal of an educational pattern that had characterized America's early years of growth, European as well as Third World students increasingly came to America's medical schools and laboratories to learn the elements of modern medicine. And, as the postwar United States continued to be thought of abroad both as a land of opportunity and as an asylum for victims of political oppression, it continued to benefit medically from the "brain drain." For other countries this meant a frequently crippling outflow of large numbers of their most talented and best trained scientists, physicians, and intellectuals. In the United States, however, such individuals quickly became useful in the medical institutions and laboratories. As such, they added not a little to the sophistication of America's medical community, helping erase lingering traces of earlier provincialism and fertilizing the health professions in ways that were productive. Above all, they became virtually indispensable in carrying out the routine measures needed to cope with disease in the fast-changing American habitats.

New Patterns of Disease and Health
in American Habitats

Even as considerable energy and resources went into helping other countries with health problems after World War II, the United States continued to have its own full share of sickness and disability. Although the impact of postwar disease was far greater in some habitats and on certain population groups than on others, most types of illness tended to affect the country as a whole. Taken together, moreover, the pervasive extent or seemingly intractable nature of certain of these afflictions made for an increasingly pessimistic popular outlook as the century progressed.

On the favorable side, a significant number of the most destructive diseases of the past had, by 1945, virtually disappeared from the American scene. Among these were yellow fever, scurvy, cholera, pellagra, malaria, smallpox, and some of the ordinary childhood diseases. Moreover, almost as modern epidemiologists watched, the discovery of new medications together with the application of quality medical care combined, during the mid-century decades, to bring about significant reductions in the incidence of additional major diseases: tuberculosis, pneumonia, influenza, childbed fever, mental disease, infant diarrheas, venereal disease, and others. To some extent, the disappearance or decline of these afflictions seemed to clear the way for other maladies in the national consciousness. As such, newer diseases became dominant in the hygienic and medical environment of America's mid-century habitats. In at least one large area of concern, the very successes of science, medicine, and the affluent society led directly, in the United States as elsewhere during this period, to new social and disease problems. These were the problems associated with the rapid increase in the numbers of the aged. This phenomenon meant, above all, a vast increase not in acute infectious diseases but in the incidence of the degenerative diseases of old age: cancer, heart and vascular system diseases, kidney disorders, stroke, and other organ failures. It also meant large new demands on hospital facilities, health insurance systems, and welfare programs. The diseases of old age could in many cases be alleviated or arrested by "high-tech" medicine. But for the aged person and his family, the new periods of longevity seemed all too often to be marked by pain, helplessness, and reliance on medications than by any substantially extended enjoyment of life.

Another large area of concern at mid-century was the plight of those of all classes whose mental well-being was impaired, whether by disease or circumstances. Public health and hospital registers had long since made it clear that, even in "normal" times, people suffered from psychoses, phobias, depressions, neuroses, and other disabling mental disorders. While a remarkable rate of improvement in these illnesses was achieved during this period by new therapies, there remained a large and often conspicuous residue of mentally sick people who continued to need care. Among these individuals were significant numbers who, for various reasons, were unable to cope with the manifold crises, fears, insecurities, or traumas of mid-twentieth-century life.

The onset of the nuclear age was a particularly potent source of anxiety for the healthy as well as for the ill. In addition to stirring up widespread generalized fears of nuclear war, the age spawned specific new public health problems that became matters of official and public concern, particularly following the reporting of radiation injuries after nuclear testing and with the occasional occurrence of accidents at nuclear power plants. To be sure, science quickly found important applications for atomic knowledge in medicine, among them the diagnostic use of radioactive isotopes. On the whole, however, the people of the United States tended to view the products of the atomic age more as curses on mankind than as sources of well-being.

Another area of concern for post–World War II Americans was the continuing threat of epidemic diseases. True, cholera, yellow fever, and some of the other older infectious menaces seemed to have retreated to their historic loci of endemicity in Asia and Africa, while the Public Health Service kept an eye on them through the various world-wide reporting mechanisms. However, these precautions could not totally dispel the apprehensions that such diseases continued to stir up, given the ease of making contacts in that age of far-flung international trade and tourism.

Meanwhile, considerable public and scientific concern was produced during this period by a number of actual outbreaks of potent new epidemic diseases or unpredictable modifications of old ones. These included several damaging pandemics of influenza in its various forms—Asian flu in 1957, Hong Kong flu in 1968, and Russian flu in 1978—as well as the mysterious but relatively restricted legionnaires' disease of 1976. Another late-twentieth-century cause of uneasiness has been the outbreak of Lyme disease that began in the northeastern states during the 1980s, the steady diffusion of which has served as a sharp reminder of the important continuing roles of animal hosts and insect vectors in the spread of human infections.

Far more alarming than any of the other epidemics has been the sudden onslaught of AIDS, beginning around 1980. AIDS spread extremely rapidly, at first particularly among homosexuals and intravenous drug users, and with a shocking rate of mortality among its victims. The general terror provoked by the disease has prompted many individuals to abandon the freewheeling sexual practices that were so prevalent earlier in the period. It has also led governments and foundations to subsidize a massive research program in the country's laboratories. However, despite these efforts, no effective medication or preventive serum had been found for the condition prior to the end of 1990.

A final devastating disease is substance addiction. On the one hand, despite reports of some decline in alcohol consumption, alcoholism has remained widespread and as destructive as ever, physically and socially. At the same time, addiction from other drugs suddenly burst its relatively modest pre–World War II bounds, from being a largely individualized disease, or at least one presumed to be limited in scope, to one that spread dismayingly through schools, playgrounds, and entire communities. Propelled by high profit incentives, "pushers" have sold their drugs and created new addicts through local distribution networks. Government and community responses of the 1980s to this demoralizing evil focused heavily on education, along with some efforts to punish drug dealers and the multiplication of detoxification programs and other centers for care of the addicted.

Whatever the gravity of the problems associated with drug addiction, AIDS, or the occasional epidemic of influenza, it appears that people in post–World War II America have not, as a whole, been any more beleaguered by menacing diseases than many earlier generations were. In fact, by the 1980s it was observable that 85 percent of the population, a larger preponderance of the American people than ever before, were living in circumstances that in most respects were favorable to maintaining ordinary good health. These are individuals whose incomes have kept them sufficiently above the poverty level to allow them to enjoy, at least to some extent, the products of America's exceptional bounty. During the postwar decades, these benefits, which by then included substantial health and medical services, became very widely distributed throughout all areas of the country. As such, they tended to minimize some of the hygienic differences between Americans' traditional habitats, i.e., the transient, rural, small town, and urban environments. Or rather, such differences now seemed to be more often based in economics than in geographical and population distribution.

By mid-century, therefore, most Americans were able to pay for needed medicines and health care and were able to provide themselves and their families with health insurance. In addition, with the country's extensive networks of good roads, telephones, and other modes of rapid transportation and communication, most were able to have reasonably ready access to the spreading hospitals, clinics, rescue systems, and other medical care facilities in or near their communities. To be sure, in practice, small towns and rural areas often experienced great continuing difficulty in retaining their physicians, other health care professionals, and even hospitals, while urban and suburban areas generally attracted more than their share.

Nevertheless, in all areas, most Americans were able, by the 1950s and 1960s, to sustain a relatively high quality of life, one which was reflected in their declining morbidity rates and their increasing longevity. They were generally able, at the least, to afford an adequate standard of housing, sufficient food and other necessaries, and some educational and leisure opportunities. Meanwhile, virtually all organized communities of any size by then were normally able to provide most of their citizens with a full range of public sanitary services including a pure water supply, effective sewage disposal, regular garbage and trash collection, and more or less clean streets. Improvements in technology even enabled isolated mid-century rural residents and farmers of any means to have the benefits of indoor plumbing and hygienic sanitary facilities.

While many members of post–World War II American society tended to boast about their generally high quality of life, they were increasingly forced to acknowledge the lamentable health conditions and resources of an all too sizeable minority, those individuals who lived near or below the poverty level. As late as 1987, one in five American children were born into families that were in that category. The mortality rate among American infants was the highest among twenty leading industrialized nations. Estimates suggest, moreover, that some 30 million individuals still have no health insurance coverage, private or public, while another 30 million lack such protection for long periods each year.

The medically disadvantaged have been found wherever economic or other personal misfortune prevailed or where social inequity stood in the way of people's betterment. Sometimes large numbers of them have lived together in separate habitats that were strongly defined by race or occupation. But the numbers also have included numerous anonymous individuals in every section of the country.

In the middle and late twentieth century, as earlier, large segments of the disadvantaged, generally homeless and virtually penniless, eventually gravitated to the transient habitat. There, lacking the resources of the age's numerous successful salesmen, consultants, and other well-paid travelers, they have experienced all of the worst features of this habitat and few of its advantages. Particularly numerous among them have been the usual derelicts, chronic alcoholics, and drug addicts, the unemployed, and runaways. But there also have been large new numbers of individuals from broken homes, patients turned out of mental hospitals and other institutions, failed farmers or white-collar workers, and others unable to cope with modern society. For all of them, the wandering life in or between cities, with little and irregular food, with sporadic medical attention, and with nights spent in public shelters, on city grates, in alleys, or under bridges, is as detrimental to health in the affluent twentieth century as such life has ever been.

Only slightly better healthwise has been the habitat of another large class of transients, the migrant farmworkers employed in various sections of the country. Generally poorly paid and overworked, such workers characteristically have been housed in hygienically marginal barracks, with little access to organized medicine or public health clinics. Working with dangerous equipment and exposed to high concentrations of the pesticides used on crops, such workers have long had one of the highest death rates in the country. Despite the efforts of health officials, legislators, union leaders, and others, improvements in the health environment have proved painfully slow in coming for this group. Equally at risk with respect to health have been the inhabitants of the twentieth-century urban ghettoes, most of them blacks and recent immigrants in poor economic circumstances. From a sanitary viewpoint, these sections of America's cities rank little better than the worst nineteenth-century slums. Alleviative measures, periodically proposed by city planners, administrators, politicians, and reformers, have been notoriously inadequate and all too often become monuments to civic neglect and failure. For the mid-and late-twentieth-century ghetto family, the obtaining of the barest minimum of housing, clothing, and food has become ever more difficult with the steady rise of prices. Similarly, the cost of health insurance and most private health care has rapidly climbed out of reach of the poor, leaving them dependent upon overburdened and understaffed public clinics and welfare institutions. Whatever medical attention the ghetto dwellers have managed to obtain has been far from enough, certainly not enough to prevent some of the highest sickness and mortality rates in the nation, particularly among children.

By the post–World War II period, nearly half of the native American or Indian population—in 1970 the total was around 790,000—also lived in urban areas, the remainder mostly on reservations under conditions that were little better. Obviously far from extinction, the race had renovated itself remarkably since its demographic low point of a century earlier. But for a large proportion, life continued to be mean, desperate, and unhealthful. As a group they have been among the most deprived in the nation, ranking at the bottom in income, education, employment, and health. Seventy percent are estimated to live in substandard housing, with levels of nutrition and hygiene that are correspondingly low. Over the years, clinics and other medical care facilities have been provided to the larger reservation groups by governments and charitable bodies, but these have consistently been far from adequate. Throughout the period, for the reservation populations at least, tuberculosis has continued to be a serious problem, infant mortality has been nearly 50 percent higher than the national rate, and the average age at death has been some 30–35 percent lower than that of the nation as a whole.

While poverty has had devastating effects on the health of many post–World War II Americans, certain developments associated predominantly with prosperity have posed new threats to health and quality of life in virtually every geographical area or habitat. The continued multiplication of people has led to increasing compactness of the urban and suburban habitats, with all that implies for sanitation and the spread of diseases. Meanwhile, the economic expansion that went along with the increase of population—the accelerated exploitation of natural resources, the paving of lands for roads and shopping malls, the transforming of farms and forests into new suburbs, and the filling up of cities with new densities of high-rise buildings—all have made for a marked deterioration of the familiar physical environment. For many, the quality of human life has been diminished by the killing off of the flora and fauna, by the great gashes cut into the agricultural and forest land, by the often uncontrolled spread of buildings into open spaces. But, the most profound effects on health in every habitat have been those brought about by the country's runaway industrialism.

By the mid-century decades, a new and sometimes upgraded generation of industrial installations of various kinds—extractive, manufacturing, transportation, agricultural—dotted the landscape in every section of the country. While many still occupied sites that were ugly, dirty, and unsanitary, other firms had built attractive new buildings, installed quieter and more efficient machinery, and eliminated some of the grosser modes by which their wastes had contaminated the air, water, or soil. At the same time, increasingly constrained by governmental regulations to give greater attention to industrial hazards and health, almost all firms had installed at least the required minimum of safety devices, while the larger also provided health and rest facilities, nurses, and physicians. However, there continued to be serious violations of plant safety and neglect of worker health. As late as mid-century, for example, the byssinosis or brown lung of cotton factory workers continued to receive little attention.

Even more serious have been the effects produced on the postwar environment and on the health of the larger society by the processes and products of industrialism. Particularly conspicuous and devastating is the loss of life and limb caused by automobiles and trucks; cancer resulting from exposure to asbestos; the effects of acid rain; destructive diseases produced by deposits of toxic wastes into waterways and landfills, by tobacco products, pesticides, the gross atmospheric contaminations produced by internal combustion engines and the sprays from aerosol cans. The century has had a proliferation of concerned calls for new controls to protect Americans' health and habitats from further devastation along these lines. However, in the United States as abroad, nagging doubts are being aired as to man's ability to act promptly enough to ensure his survival on a polluted planet.

Amalgamation: The New Medical Establishment as Colossus

However alarming the mounting toll of ills associated with industrialism, and however baffling the period's varied other major diseases, members of America's mainline medical community have felt well able to cope with the situation. In fact, even if their ability to prevent disease is still limited, for the first time individuals belonging to the organized medical professions and their allies at least consider themselves equipped with the knowledge, resources, institutions, and personnel to effectively alleviate or cure a large portion of this sickness. And for those associated with every segment of the expanding regular medical enterprise, the perception of widespread scientific and therapeutic successes has done much to strengthen professional confidence.

During the early decades of the twentieth century, the body of practicing physicians represented by the American Medical Association (A.M.A.) had assumed the predominant position in the nation's medical scene. Other components—the medical research community, medical industry, the hospital enterprise, and the federal government health community—originally played essentially supportive roles. As they expanded their activities and institutions, however, these latter components began to play larger roles and in some instances to challenge the leadership of the A.M.A. This trend was accelerated by the requirements of World War II, which dictated new kinds of relationships between the components. By the postwar period, therefore, a revised nationwide medical system was largely in place, one that involved a new high degree of interlocking interest and activity between the various large components. In fact, the functions of these components became so interdependent as to constitute a vast new medical establishment, one that far eclipsed in size, scope, and impact the one that had flourished earlier in the century.

One effect of the emergence of large new components in the establishment, each with its own interests, was a significant redistribution of medical power. In particular, by the post–World War II decades, the A.M.A. was being forced to share its medical influence with the other interest groups. Increasing parts of that power now gravitated to scientific, industrial, and insurance groups; to the medical press and consumer organizations; to foundations and to academia; and above all to government agencies. Other societies representing large health professions—bodies such as the American Pharmaceutical Association, the American Hospital Association, the American Nurses' Association, the American Dental Association, and the American

College of Surgeons, as well as organizations representing the powerful medical specialties—also carried far more weight than before with legislators and policy formulators. This is not to suggest that the A.M.A., with its thousands of members, was no longer a highly potent force. On the contrary, it continued to represent its members effectively, extended its services, and refined its formidable lobbying activities. But its generally conservative political positions could no longer be assumed to prevail with little opposition. More and more, medical policymaking became a process of seeking compromises through extended discussion, education, and politicking by the various medical interest groups, each with large constituencies and sophisticated public relations apparatus.

Along with these shifts in medical power, the nature of orthodox medical practice in the United States itself changed rapidly and drastically. As penicillin, the antibiotics, and other new drugs came on the market, along with antipolio vaccine, DPT, and other new vaccines or sera, postwar physicians almost overnight found themselves finally able to substantially influence the course of numerous of their patients' diseases. They filled their offices with ever more sophisticated instruments and relied ever more routinely on the laboratory for many of their diagnoses. At some point during these years, particularly in large cities, they ceased making house calls. And, at about the same time, impressed by the World War II successes of the Kaiser-Permanente health organization and group specialist practice in the services, many physicians began joining together in group practice, quickly bringing respectability to what had been one of the nineteenth-century medical establishment's principal bugaboos.

Not least of the various postwar changes was the accelerated decline and threatened extinction of the general practitioner—of that all-too-often ineffective yet indispensable species whose individual members had epitomized both the best and the worst about medicine for generations of Americans. Pushing traditional general practice relentlessly aside, medical specialization came into full flower as a logical result of the splintering of modern scientific and medical knowledge. The phenomenon was particularly conspicuous in the cities and suburbs, where the new accumulations of doctors' buildings and shopping malls were rapidly dominated by the offices of physicians devoted variously to urology, gerontology, cardiology, pediatrics, neurology, otolaryngology, and the numerous other medical specialties and subspecialties. Backing each specialty across the country were the accumulations of societies, journals, and increasingly influential specialty boards. Typically, but not a little incongruously, when attempts were made to revive general practice by training and certifying interested new physicians, it was proposed to categorize the latter as specialists of family medicine.

As the physician's practice changed, so did that of other mainline health-related professions. Twentieth-century dentists, like other professionals, increasingly divided up into subspecialties. The introduction of new equipment and materials made their work increasingly rapid and effective, while the reduction of pain through continued improvement in anesthetics made going to the dentist infinitely more appealing for the public than it had been in earlier generations.

The century's pharmacists, in the meantime, while also progressively well organized and trained, experienced considerable change in the nature and scope of their profession. Outside of hospitals, their research roles increasingly passed to academic or commercial chemists and pharmacologists, while their role in the manufacture of drugs came to be almost entirely assumed by large corporations. In turn, the compounding of medicines became a steadily more standardized process, while drug retailing has frequently become only one department among many in large variety stores.

In certain social respects, the character of the country's health-related practices has been deeply affected by mid-century civil rights movements. Women had already gained at least nominal access to most medical schools, societies, and hospitals. However, the numbers of women in medicine and the other health professions remained small during the early postwar decades. Womens' rights groups seeking to increase the proportion of women physicians thus began focusing increased attention on pay differentials and other forms of discrimination said to have been used against them. In turn, nurses became progressively more vocal in opposing what they identified as the traditional chauvinism and authoritarianism of male physicians and more active in working for equitable roles in the hospitals.

Access for black physicians and medical students to the professional institutions of the white medical establishment, meanwhile, remained highly limited in many parts of the country at the end of World War II. Little improvement in this situation was achieved until the enactment of equal rights legislation at mid-century. At the same time, blacks were only gradually admitted to positions where they could gain recognition in the medical sciences. Conspicuous twentieth-century exceptions were Eugene Just for his research in cytology, William Hinton for contributions to the treatment of syphilis, and Charles Drew for his work on blood transfusion. Similarly, any significant modification or termination of the separate and unequal hospital arrangements for blacks, particularly in the southern states, had to wait until after the Supreme Court's mid-century decisions ending segregation.

Nationwide, further hospital construction and improvement was stimulated in the postwar decades by new sources of funds, particularly those provided by the federal Hill-Burton Act of 1946. This act aimed at establishing hospitals in smaller cities, towns, and rural areas that had not previously had such facilities, as well as renovating and adding on to existing institutions. With these new facilities physicians almost everywhere were now able to send their seriously ill patients to hospitals. There, high caliber nursing care could usually be taken for granted, while large staffs of medical specialists and technicians utilizing elaborate and expensive diagnostic and therapeutic devices were on call. The larger institutions developed intensive care units and trauma centers, while outpatient services were greatly expanded everywhere.

While it had been evolving some since early in the century, the postwar general hospital has been increasingly marked by change. Private nonprofit hospitals have continued to make up the largest proportion of such institutions, though profit-making hospitals are increasing in number and governmental institutions continue to be important. As a general thing, hospitals have come to be better organized than they were in 1940, and more often run by professional administrators. Many have become parts of extended hospital systems or corporate networks. The private hospital has been progressively shaped by the financial imperatives of its links with health insurance programs and government medical aid. In the process, as Stevens points out, the private nonprofit hospital has increasingly directed its services toward middle-class and upper-class patients and has gradually lost much of its traditional character as a community charity. Government-run public institutions, by default, have taken on more of the charity patients, while they have also been left to provide a disproportionate share of the hospitalization of the chronically ill, all those requiring long-term treatment and rehabilitation. The private hospitals, in short, have typically come to focus mainly on acute problems and emergency situations. They feature intensive surgery and therapy utilizing highly sophisticated technology, and normally provide only short-term stays in the hospital for the patients. As "state-of-the-art" institutions, the general hospitals have become, more than ever before, the essential central elements in the health care provided in American communities. However, the future of many of these facilities, particularly those in small towns and rural areas, has become increasingly problematic, above all because of high costs.

Mid-twentieth-century developments also include drastic alter-
ations in the extent and nature of certain kinds of special hospitals.
Private clinics for particular disease conditions have flourished more
than ever before, while custodial nursing homes for the aged have
become big businesses. In some communities, hospices have appeared in response to the demand for humane care of the terminally
ill. On the other side of the coin, the country's far-flung network of
tuberculosis sanatoria disappeared almost overnight with the coming
of antibiotic therapy in the 1950s, while the scattered infectious disease hospitals were also phased out. Shortly after this, a large and
controversial exodus, stimulated partly by civil rights advocates and
mandated by judicial decisions, began from mental hospitals. This
deinstitutionalizing of mental disease has undoubtedly released
many patients to newly productive lives, but it has also left many
others confused, homeless, and vulnerable where alternative community support mechanisms have failed.

While an ever-increasing overall proportion of twentieth-century
America's sick people have been treated in hospitals, individual patients have not necessarily experienced a steady bettering of physical
conditions and support in those institutions. To be sure, the bedside
routine of nurses and orderlies became more highly organized, but
efficiency often brought a decline in the personal attention that patients craved. The advance of technology, meanwhile, added a new
arsenal of sophisticated diagnostic, operative, and therapeutic procedures to the hospitals' capabilities, and from which patients came to
have a very high expectation of cure and elimination of pain. However, to gain some measure of these benefits, patients frequently
found that they had to put up with a highly uncomfortable maze of
wires, hoses, catheters, straps, and monitors that enveloped them in
the sickbed. As in earlier generations, most contemporary physicians
visiting the sickbed are undoubtedly concerned about how their patients are feeling. But all to often their attention seems to focus more
on the workings of the various devices than on the comfort of the
patient.

The late-twentieth-century patient, facing the possibility of death
from a malignant cancer, AIDS, organ failure, or some other condition, has a variety of nurses, specialists, and technicians, as well as
his or her surgeon and general practitioner, to talk with about illnesses, pains, fears, and prospects for recovery. But for many, most
of whatever spiritual comfort and encouragement they receive comes
from the hospital volunteers and chaplains, along with the visits of
family, clergy, and friends. And ultimately family members, who are
removed from direct physical care roles as long as the patient remains

in the hospital, resume those burdens as well as soon as the patient is discharged.

In the largest and best equipped general hospitals, as well as some of the others, postwar surgery has spawned what the public sees as a new body of medical "supermen," operators with all the audacity and dramatics of their predecessors from earlier generations, but backed by a far more complex and sometimes controversial technology. Some of them pushed such specialties as brain and gastrointestinal surgery forward to remarkable new heights. Others claimed attention as developers of artificial organs and performers of transplants from patient to patient. A widespread new vogue of plastic surgery took off on the wave of postwar prosperity. And cataract surgery, with the successful introduction of plastic lens inserts in the late 1970s, changed overnight from a harrowing and uncertain procedure to a relatively painless and routine one, with some million and a half operations annually. Particularly appealing to the postwar public has been heart surgery, a procedure that hardly existed anywhere in 1940 but by the 1960s was becoming an everyday occurrence. Propelled first of all by a series of headlining heart transplants in the United States and abroad, the specialty also has attracted much attention with its experimental artificial hearts. But it came into its own with the successful development of the pacemaker and the spectacular evolution of the heart bypass operation as a surgical routine.

The most advanced twentieth-century hospitals have developed increasingly close relationships with affiliated medical schools. In many such cases, huge medical center complexes incorporate more than one hospital, together with schools of medicine, dentistry, nursing, public health, pharmacy, and other medical professions. While a number of new medical schools emerged after World War II, the competition for admissions has remained intense. Not a few unsuccessful candidates have turned to foreign medical schools, particularly in Latin America. At the same time, the postwar shortage of physicians attracted considerable numbers of foreign medical graduates to the United States. Some of these were able to take hospital staff positions almost immediately. Others, however, had to invest in several further years of specialized study in order to obtain their American qualifications.

By mid-century, American medical schools, as well as teaching hospitals, for the most part had long since shaped themselves after the Johns Hopkins model, in which research tended to be the dominant basic component. To some in the medical profession, the emphasis on research has steadily come to be an increasingly mixed blessing. For such individuals, the situation is one which, by emphasizing the production of new knowledge, downplays the importance of applying already existing knowledge in the cure of sick patients. As such the schools' effectiveness in preparing ordinary medical practitioners seems to have diminished. Despite this critique, however, throughout the postwar period the mystique of research and the ready availability of funds for investigation have remained dominant considerations for a majority of medical faculty members and students alike.

America's early-twentieth-century regular medical establishment had indeed benefited enormously by linking its fortunes to the outlook and methods of laboratory science. And, through subsequent decades of this century, the establishment had no reason to change, for the postwar biomedical sciences were more creative and productive than ever before. Research had not only become the preferred activity of a considerable segment of the nation's best trained medical doctors, but the pursuit of numerous other professional scientists and far larger numbers of technicians. By 1940 America's biomedical research enterprise was already marked by an impressive and numerous assortment of laboratories located in medical schools, hospitals, pharmaceutical firms, university science departments, independent institutes, health departments, armed forces installations, and other agencies. But during the postwar decades, thanks to an unprecedented infusion of new funds from government, the foundations, and other sources, research facilities have grown still more, both in number and in size.

In the respective institutions research of various kinds, basic as well as applied or clinical, has often been carried out under mandates to attack one or another "categorical" medical condition: heart disease, old age, mental illness, stroke, arthritis, or above all, cancer, plus such currently alarming infections as influenza, Lyme disease, and AIDS. In America's postwar laboratories, the research ranks were originally filled predominantly by individuals trained as physiologists, chemists and biochemists, pathologists, and microbiologists. But as these individuals pursued their work, often with international collaborators, they helped open up various new scientific fields. The spread of the electron microscope and other new items of equipment, for example, helped lead to a take-off in virology and protozoology. Nuclear development gave an enormous impetus to molecular biology and biophysics generally, and the breaking of the genetic code opened up vast new horizons both for medical genetics and for immunology. In fact, virtually every area of biomedical science, not excluding the behavioral sciences, has changed almost beyond recognition during this period.

The upsurge in the sciences was accompanied and stimulated by a substantial postwar increase in the numbers of individuals with advanced competence in mathematics and statistics. And the research processes were even further revolutionized, virtually overnight, by the rapid introduction of computers into the laboratories. The computer has also made possible the establishment of elaborately automated medical and scientific communication systems. Particularly significant has been the National Library of Medicine's computerized national network, introduced in the 1960s, for rapid retrieval and dissemination of the world's biomedical literature, a system with thousands of outlets at laboratories, hospitals, and universities around the United States, as well as abroad.

Expanding fully as rapidly as the research enterprise in postwar America have been the country's diverse medical industries. In fact, as a component of big business, medical industry has become an ever more conspicuous aspect of the medical enterprise in society. Innovative in its technology and aggressive in seeking profits, its personnel and products have been increasingly important in fueling the upsurge of medical research as well as in making the results of research available to the medical care professions and the public.

Two kinds of health industries have become particularly prominent. One large segment, comprising the pharmaceutical corporations, continued the vigorous growth and international expansion that had started during and after World War I. By the 1950s the operations of this type of industry included not only the manufacture, distribution, and promotion of every kind of drug or medication, but also research and development of new products on a large scale.

Another large cluster of health industries includes the manufacturers and suppliers of medical equipment of all kinds. Such firms proliferated noticeably during and after World War II. They have included, for instance, makers of and dealers in highly sophisticated and costly diagnostic apparatus, of laboratory instruments and materials, of hospital and home care supplies and therapeutic devices. The individual products range from lenses, hearing aids, and pacemakers, to dialysis systems, office files, ambulances, and anesthesia monitors.

Many postwar developments have added to the growing image of medicine as a business operation. Advertising in professional medical journals and the general press alike has highlighted the intense competition within the various medical industries. Individuals, meanwhile, have increasingly come to finance their doctors' bills and hospital expenses through large pre-paid health insurance organizations or other intermediary bodies. And above all, in every type of medical institution—hospitals, laboratories, medical schools—administrative tasks have become ever more pressing and prominent. Record-keeping and report-making has expanded along with the meetings of medical committees, while fund raisers and grant management officials have become indispensable.

In back of much of this new administrative activity lie the programs and requirements of the federal government. In fact, Washington has proved to be behind almost every aspect of America's postwar medical revolution. This massive expansion of federal influence in health-related matters has been no accident. Eight years of the New Deal, followed by five years of war mobilization, accustomed Americans to look increasingly to a strong central government to meet their needs and to organize the various strands of their society. Moreover, postwar social expectations were high and long-deferred or partially fulfilled medical and health improvements proved to have remarkably high priority among the items on the national agenda.

The outcome was an unprecedented spate of federal health legislation, starting immediately after World War II and continuing almost unabated up into the 1980s. Existing federal health agencies and their institutions were consolidated and strengthened, while new ones came into being. The mandating of specific new programs gave these agencies and their institutions enormously increased influence in the various areas of medicine. This power was exerted partly through direct health activities and regulatory requirements. But it was even more broadly diffused through the distribution of federal funds to local governments and private institutions, along with the formulation and management of health policy regarding their use.

Setting the pace as early as 1946 was the passage of the Hill-Burton Act, providing assistance for the financing of hospitals. Following this, during the next decade, legislation gave increased status and focus to the missions of the Public Health Service, Food and Drug Administration, and other health-related components of the Federal Security Agency. After 1953 the latter agency was upgraded and given cabinet status as the Department of Health, Education and Welfare, precursor of today's Department of Health and Human Services.

Of major importance during the postwar decades was a new congressional interest in medical research. Building on the Public Health Service's old Hygienic Laboratory and the more recent National Cancer Institute (1937), Congress passed a succession of acts that gave shape to what ultimately became the National Institutes of Health (NIH), with its cluster of research institutes focusing on major disease entities. In its laboratories NIH carried out both basic and applied research on a host of biomedical problems. At the same time, through grants, fellowships, and contracts, it stimulated and influenced the course of research elsewhere. By such mechanisms, immense sums of money were funneled, throughout this period, into America's hospitals, medical schools, university science departments, and other institutions in support of research and of the training of medical scientists. In the process, the country's biomedical scientists were everywhere brought into close relationships with the federal government, while the character of America's institutions of higher learning as well as of its local health agencies has been profoundly altered.

As Strickland and other historians have pointed out, Congress's enthusiastic support of medical research diverted many during this time from the pursuit of effective and comprehensive federal health care provisions. In 1965, however, among the conspicuous reforms of the "Great Society" era, Congress did enact legislation that brought the United States substantially closer to a form of national health insurance. This included passage of the Medicare Act for the aged and the Medicaid Act for the poor. Attempts also continued to overhaul the nation's health care system even more drastically by extending provisions of these acts to the whole population. Failing achievement of that end, the most pressing legislative and medical concern during the subsequent years has been to try to control the crushing costs of Medicare and Medicaid, though that effort has had little success. During the same period, however, Congress has continued to expand the scope of federal health authority. Most conspicuously this has resulted in the creation of new national health programs and agencies aimed at the betterment of occupational and industrial health and the improvement of environmental health conditions.

With these new programs added to the old, the federal government has exercised a steadily increasing measure of influence over the quality and extent of public health activities at other levels, though state and local agencies have retained much control over implementation and everyday operations. It has provided funds for water supply and sewage-filtration systems as well as for maternal and infant health care clinics. It coordinates and supplements measures for surveillance and control of infectious diseases. It has expanded its efforts to standardize and improve drugs and vaccines and to ensure food safety. And it has pulled together and analyzed local health statistics of all kinds to determine national trends and needs. Such statistics contributed significantly to one of the Public Health Service's most controversial and important twentieth-century health initiatives, the Surgeon-General's early 1960s study of the effects of smoking. The study confirmed the close causative relationship of smoking with cancer, as well as with other dread diseases. And as such, it provided the impetus for nationwide educational programs and legislative acts which, within two decades, remarkably reduced the long-time American addiction to tobacco.

The exercise of these and other new forms of health-related authority during the post–World War II decades has helped the federal government to assume an ever more intimate and conspicuous involvement in virtually all the workings of the nation's mainline medical system, curative and preventive. Scientists and administrators in government agencies have taken on ever larger new roles as regulators, coordinators, and financiers, not only of federal activities but of state and local programs, and in many ways those of other components of the enlarged medical establishment as well. In the process, they have also come into progressively closer relationships, direct and indirect, with individual Americans in their search for health.

By mid-century the proliferating institutions and activities of the establishment—professional, therapeutic, industrial, scientific, and governmental—were touching the lives and affecting the well-being of nearly every citizen. Americans utilized these facilities on a large scale, and by and large they seemed to look forward to obtaining more such benefits. They welcomed the improved diagnoses, the high degree of relief from pain, the widely successful therapies for many of their most feared ailments. And yet, as the system expanded and became more complex, more and more persons became dissatisfied with or critical of some part of its workings.

To a certain extent, this discontent may reflect the build-up of a generalized sense of nostalgia for the old horse and buggy doctor and the simpler medical world that he represented. More serious, however, are the antagonisms that many post–World War II Americans, like their forebears, have harbored against unfeeling medical institutions and authorities, together with the resentments they have built up with respect to the regular physicians' privileges and perceived elitism. There seems to have been a constant reservoir of hostility directed against such things as the increased commercialism of hospitals, the high fees of specialists, and the profiteering of some physicians, as well as the corporate greed of some pharmaceutical firms and medical equipment manufacturers. At the same time, many laypeople have simply been overwhelmed by the size, complexity, and bureaucratic features of many medical institutions or offended by the impersonal or tactless attitudes of personnel in them. And numerous other individuals are fearful of some of the research going on in medical institutions, for instance in such threatening areas as genetic engineering.

Among the more active critics of mainline medicine have been members of groups that revived and extended some of the most deeply felt medical protests of earlier generations. Antivaccinationists, for instance, reappeared after World War II in opposition to certain governmental inoculation programs, both on general principles and because the programs seemed to have inadequate safeguards. Other groups have sporadically rallied against proposals for public water fluoridation, most often on grounds that they were socialistic. And more potent than any of these groups has been the fast-growing and highly motivated membership of the new generation of animal rights advocates. These are individuals who, among other issues, protest against what they perceived as an increase of cruelties inflicted on laboratory animals in the nation's biomedical research installations.

Less publicized but probably the most numerous and anguished of the protests are those that have to do with the modern age's therapeutic practices. All too many late-twentieth-century patients have complained about unneeded surgery or being put on excessive drug regimens. Large numbers of women have rallied against the overmedicalization of childbirth and explored means of recapturing more meaningful roles for themselves in the experience. In the course of hospital treatment, individuals frequently find the high-tech procedures not only intimidating but frequently more painful than their maladies. And families of the seriously ill have often been appalled by the heroic measures that are increasingly taken to prolong life. As the Congressional Office of Technology Assessment reported in the mid-1980s, "while hospitals were once feared as 'places to die' because so little could be done to avert death, some people now fear hospitals as places to die because so much can be done."

While twentieth-century individuals all too often have been able to do little about such medical grievances, a variety of organized lay bodies have sought to represent the public interests that were involved. Consumer groups, senior citizens organizations, churches, the press, and feminist and health activist associations, all at times have been effective foci of opposition to specific medical practices. And together they exert considerable pressure for more humane medical environments in their respective communities.

The issues that concern these lay bodies have been equally troubling to many mid-century health professionals. Solutions for the various complaints of medical users, patients and their families, are conscientiously sought for in the ongoing discussions of medical soci ety meetings and special committees. Individual professionals, meanwhile, especially after 1960, have shown new interest in the philosophical and ethical ramifications of the various medical procedures and sciences. Medical schools even introduced courses on medical ethics into their crowded curricula.

While these activities within the professional medical community have presumably been motivated by genuine social concern, there were also undoubted considerations of self-interest. The dissatisfactions of patients, families, or advocacy groups with specific aspects of regular therapy could, some feared, easily grow into a more general lack of public confidence in mainline medicine. And this, in turn, might conceivably lead to renewed interest in and even defections to alternative health concepts or therapies. Incongruous or even grotesque as such an eventuality has surely appeared to many of the devotees of modern scientific medicine, it still remains not just a possibility but a reality in certain ways.

The Persistent Search for Health beyond Orthodox Medicine

By the middle of the twentieth century, members of the regular medical profession could be excused for supposing that their system of therapy was all that mankind required, and that the ordinary layperson's long-standing desire to retain a variety of medical options had become a thing of the past. For some regular physicians, the scientifically based procedures now at their disposal seemed to have rendered hygienic pursuits virtually unnecessary if not archaic. Moreover, the few remaining therapeutic sects, in addition to being annoyances to the orthodox, appeared to them to be anachronistic and slightly amusing artifacts in the modern medical world, and as such they seemed certain to disappear at an early date. As it happened, however, both organized and informal irregular therapeutic groups have continued to flourish during the prosperous post–World War II decades, while the appurtenances of hygienic living, also largely outside organized medicine, have remained as important to individual citizens as ever before, and often more so.

It should not have been surprising to anyone that certain organized therapeutic sects continued to exist in mid-twentieth-century America as successful and conspicuous alternatives to regular medicine. This is not to say that they offer the same threats to the medical establishment or play the same roles as their nineteenth-century counterparts had, as complete therapeutic systems. But they do continue to hold a strong collective appeal for individuals who mistrust or are somehow disenchanted with mainline medicine. They have appealed also to anti-authoritarian sentiments that flourish throughout society. Moreover, as earlier, they satisfy a variety of needs that regular medicine continues to neglect or ignore.

Under the protection of state licensing, therefore, both osteopathy and optometry have done well during this period. They consolidated their professional and economic positions, and even gained at least partial, if reluctant endorsement from the regular establishment, which sometimes incorporated them into mainline institutions. Chiropractic, by contrast, has proved able to flourish even without any suggestion of orthodox approval. The number of states in which it was licensed grew steadily after 1940, while the therapy enjoyed a remarkable increase in the numbers of its institutions, practitioners, and popularity with the public.

Meanwhile, certain religious bodies also continued to provide Americans with another kind of therapeutic option. On the one hand, to be sure, one of the older mental healing sects, Christian Science, experienced a decline in appeal and numbers. On the other hand, however, a rise in the number of charismatic religious leaders during the post–World War II decades signaled a substantial spread of the practice of faith healing among fundamentalist congregations.

The period also brought about the renewal or updating of certain previously widely used therapies and considerable experimentation with others, some of them exotic. To an extent this trend represented the rediscovery by trained physicians, nurses, and other regular health professionals of certain values in older styles of therapy. The participation of such professionals proved to be an essential ingredient in the rebirth of several such therapies. However, the major reason for their new successes was the widespread active interest and involvement of America's literate laypeople in the search for more personal or humane forms of treatment.

One result of this search was a modest revival of interest in homeopathy. This is a system that has remained popular abroad and one whose individualistic "infinitesimal" dosages now once more provide some Americans with welcome antidotes to the modern versions of the regulars' impersonal heroic treatment. Somewhat similarly, the mid-twentieth-century formulation of "holistic" medicine has represented a return to earlier concerns for the whole person, mental as well as physical. Still broader in extent is a renewed American popular interest in and use of herbal medicines and folk recipes. This is a phenomenon, moreover, that has been paralleled by the launching of far-flung scientific studies by ethnobotanists and pharmacologists on the medicinal properties of the remedies used around the world in indigenous cultures.

The World War II and postwar experiences of numerous Americans overseas included a certain exposure to and new understanding of Asian medical and health-related concepts or pursuits. One result was a substantial growth of interest in the psychological and physical aspects of Zen, Yoga, and Asian martial arts, and the subsequent mushrooming of classes in such subjects. Individuals in the United States also began to give added attention to the principles and practices of the age-old medical systems of the Indian subcontinent, Japan, Korea, and China. Acupuncture even came to enjoy a measure of official sanction following President Nixon's visit to China, though America's laboratories did not display much enthusiasm for conducting research on the measure. By contrast, however, it came to have unexpectedly wide popular favor in the United States, especially through the emergence of acupuncture clinics wherever substantial communities of Vietnamese and other new Asian immigrants have gathered.

However much mid- and late-twentieth-century Americans have turned for relief to practitioners of alternative therapies, native or imported, or to establishment medicine either, for that matter, they continue, as men and women always have done in times of sickness, to rely so far as possible upon their own devices. They turn to simple concoctions that had been recommended by mothers and friends. They avidly consult newspaper medical advice columns, magazine articles, pamphlets, and books. They follow the medical suggestions of radio and television advertisements. They go to drugstores far more often than they go to doctors' offices or clinics. And, in addition to whatever prescribed drugs they use, they treat themselves with greater quantities than ever of nonprescription preparations and devices. Finally, at least partly in the hope of warding off disease, they pursue various of the precepts and modes of hygiene, often with fanatical dedication and energy.

One of the accomplishments of twentieth-century American society has been to bring truly hygienic living within the reach of a large proportion of its citizens, partly as a result of the provision, throughout most of the country, of the basic public sanitary facilities and services. By mid-century, safe running water, bathrooms and kitchens with good plumbing, regular sanitary waste disposal facilities, and central heating units had become normal expectations for most people in their housing. At the same time, the ideals of good personal hygiene—cleanliness, tooth-brushing, getting regular exercise, the pursuit of moderation in diet, exposure to fresh air, and so on—more than ever had come to be taken for granted as standard parts of a generally accepted social ethic as well as individual desiderata. As in earlier generations, rudimentary health and hygiene principles were disseminated in the home, while greater detail was being provided by nurses and other health professionals. They remained important topics in the programs of elementary schools, health departments, and private agencies. But the crusading individual health reformers of the past seemed to have almost disappeared. Taking their places, the most conspicuous and vigorous post–World War II proponents of hygienic living have tended to be the agents of commerce. In the name of one or another aspects of hygiene, these agents and promoters have aggressively built and run a remarkably far-flung range of facilities and activities, though some of them are only marginally related to the actual maintenance or improvement of health.

Of these activities, the pursuit of physical exercise, individual sports, and recreation has remained for many mid-century Americans the most promising means of "keeping in condition," of maintaining their general health. New modes of accomplishing this have been added to old, and agencies public and private have joined in making them more attractive and more accessible to the individual than ever before. "Staying in shape" can be pursued indoors as well as outdoors. And, in some form or another, it now involves women as much as men and often the handicapped along with the unimpaired.

For many individuals, the modern quest for health has taken the form of a resurgent interest in weight-lifting and body-building. For others it is by participation in newly fashionable aerobic dance classes. Jogging has become a remarkably serious preoccupation for many, while systematic walking schedules and hiking have attracted other large numbers. Swimming is increasingly feasible the year around, as is tennis and handball. Canoeing, kayaking, and rafting have gained many new adherents, while recreational skiing and bicycling also have large clienteles.

Quite apart from their professional aspects, almost all of these forms of exercise and sport have been commercialized in one way or another, a process that grew with the population. The use of soaps and deodorants, for instance, was a natural and desirable by-product of exercise, and the promotion of such products was lucrative. However, the manufacture and sale of the various types of exercise equipment, accessories, and clothing—sport shoes of many kinds, sweatsuits, racquets and balls, weights, boats and paddles, skis and poles, home pools, bicycles, and so on—has yielded far greater profits, by 1985, several billion dollars annually.

Even more profitable has been the development and building of new facilities for recreation, sport, and hygiene. Country clubs and sports facilities have continued to proliferate. Resort hotels along the shore or in the mountains have been increasingly designed for year-round use, often providing a considerable variety of recreational facilities that are served as well as promoted by efficient travel enterprises. In the cities and suburbs, chains of mass-membership health clubs and gymnasiums have sprung up to facilitate and exploit the era's rage for physical culture. Widely called "spas," many bear little resemblance to the leisurely nineteenth-century therapeutic institutions of that name. Others, however, those that provide saunas, hot tubs, massages, and related features, along with their pools, represent a significant twentieth-century continuation of the balneological tradition.

While private enterprise has built and run many of the facilities that are central to modern America's pursuit of physical well-being and health, governments, despite limited budgets, also make important contributions. Local governments, attempting to keep up with community needs, continue as they can to lay out new urban parks, bike trails, and other facilities, though often they do well just to maintain existing public playgrounds, pools, and tennis courts. Similarly, federal and state agencies are equally hard put to maintain the hiking trails, campgrounds, resorts, and other recreational facilities that they operate. Moreover, there is a question of whether the public parks and wilderness areas can even continue to preserve the pure air and water, the stillnesses and wooded landscapes, and the other features that visitors often find to be therapeutic in one way or another.

Although late-twentieth-century exercise regimens sometimes have had only indirect relationships to the health of individuals, nutrition has played a steadily more direct hygienic role. Stimulated by the postwar spread of prepackaged "junk" food, for instance, together with such factors as the increased popularity of eating out at restaurants, obesity and ailments of the digestive system have appeared to be about as prevalent as at almost any earlier period. While the postwar period's regular physicians, like their predecessors, were kept busy treating such ailments, until late in the period few of them demonstrated much interest in dealing with the dietary practices of their patients or prescribing preventive therapies. However, other groups made nutrition a consistent central concern. At one level, homeopaths, herbalists, holistic practitioners, and other alternative medicine groups had always placed much stress on careful diet. And they were now joined by a sizable new generation of vegetarians. The concerns of these individuals and groups led to a proliferation of health-food stores in American cities and suburbs. Wherever they sprang up, these stores gave form to and support for the mid-century thirsts for nonestablishment, nonlaboratory, nontechnological approaches to health.

At another level of nutrition concern are the varied therapies available to overweight individuals. Many persons have been swept up in strenuous exercise binges, such as daily television exercise classes, as antidotes to the negative effects of their bad eating habits. Others undergo liposuction operations or, if they are sufficiently well-to-do, patronize so-called "fat farms." Still others undertake diets under supervision of their physicians. But for far more individuals, diets have tended to be standardized and impersonal procedures that one carried out after consulting a book or, more often, after purchasing a set of instructions through the mails from commercial entrepreneurs.

Meanwhile, at yet another level, post–World War II America has seen the work of consumer groups, home economists, dietitians, nutrition scientists, and others broaden significantly in an important joint effort to improve nutrition and dietary practices. Going beyond the public health inspection of foods, such individuals became progressively more active in pressing governments and manufacturers for the nutritional improvement and labeling of food products. They launched new dietary awareness programs in institutions and in the various media. And above all they aired recent findings of the sciences that demonstrated startlingly direct relationships of certain food components to heart disease, stroke, and other major diseases. The campaign that has been undertaken in the latter decades of the century to promote an understanding and reduction of cholesterol in diet is only one aspect of the large health education effort of these groups, one that, despite continuing controversy and uncertainty, has already led almost overnight to revolutionary new levels of lay and medical concern for nutrition.

A final aspect of the traditional realm of hygiene, that of sexual behavior, has changed in equally radical ways. At base, the post–World War II period saw a widespread repudiation of the Victorian Era's persistent belief in sexual moderation as a requisite of healthful living. In its place, the leaders of the twentieth-century's sexual revolution preached that more frequent and less inhibited sexual activity made for healthier individuals. And in the process they opened up both the public and the medical discussion of every aspect of sex. Widely cast aside were such old views as the limiting of the frequency of intercourse for optimal physical and mental health, the practice of abstaining from sex except for reproduction, the belief in the evil effects of masturbation. Taking their place has been a new appreciation of the sexual urge as a normal part of the make-up of women as well as of men. A new degree of understanding of and accommodation to homosexuality also began to be evident, though this has been set back by the onset of the AIDS scare in the 1980s.

The liberation of women and the new freedoms of sex behavior, together with the accumulations of new scientific knowledge, have made for steadily broader professional roles for physicians in sexual matters than many of them had been accustomed to play. Health professionals of all kinds, to be sure, were heartened and aided in treating venereal disease by the advent of the antibiotics and other drugs. Gynecologists have been increasingly asked to fit women with one or another of the new contraceptive devices. In turn, surgeons have been called upon to perform such operations as sex changes and breast enhancements. They are also increasingly called upon to perform operations to terminate the individual man or woman's capacity to fertilize or be fertilized. Not a few physicians, moreover, continue to perform abortions, though the social and legal status of this procedure has remained uncertain throughout the period.

The age has likewise greatly broadened social acceptance of contraception as an essential factor in sexual freedom and enjoyment, as well as in women's health and in couples' efforts to achieve economic well-being. Official policy of the Roman Catholic Church and some other religious bodies has continued to prohibit the use of birth control devices, but many individual American members of these churches have nevertheless utilized them regularly. At the same time, research in reproductive biology during this period has resulted in a considerable variety of new preventive medications and improved mechanical devices. Some, however, produced alarming and widely publicized side-effects and have had to be withdrawn from the market.

A central feature of the new era of sex hygiene has been a renewed commitment to sex education. Health agencies and birth control clinics became especially effective in distributing large quantities of pamphlets, and they have often provided speakers on the subject. Early scholarly surveys of Americans' sex habits attracted remarkably wide attention. Particularly celebrated among these were the studies of Alfred C. Kinsey in 1948 and 1953 and those of William H. Masters and Virginia E. Johnson beginning in the 1960s. These were followed by a succession of equally detailed inquiries into Americans' sex habits, with "how to" guides to happy and healthy sex ultimately acquiring the status of perennial best sellers in the nation's bookstores. Eventually, moreover, public schools in some areas again began offering sex education courses, albeit uneasily in many cases. Undoubtedly the period's most remarkable step in sex education, however, has been the vigorous promotion of condoms during the 1980s as part of the effort to control AIDS. As a result of that campaign, this device, which only a few years earlier could not be mentioned in polite society, has almost overnight gained the ultimate in modern public exposure through a combination of official and commercial advertising—in buses, in the press, and on television.

The middle- and late-twentieth-century contributors to sex hygiene, nutrition, and exercise therapy have sometimes left the impression of having gone over to America's medical establishment. Like curative medicine, these various facets of modern hygiene came to be heavily shaped in content and practice by the findings of laboratory science. They attracted and gained the active participation of increasing numbers of orthodox physicians along with laypeople and irregulars. And, as with the regular establishment, certain of hygiene's activities and products were taken over in this century by commercial and mass marketing interests. Yet, in other respects hygiene remained firmly outside the focus of mainline medicine. Most important, it has continued to be substantially at odds with the latter's curative emphasis and its professional structures. And, as such, it has kept its place as a significant ally of the persistent therapeutic sects, together with the various medical advocate groups and other elements that make up the country's nonestablishment medical world.

As in earlier generations, the components of alternative medicine thus provide Americans with important therapeutic and hygienic options. At the same time, they continue to play substantial roles as critics of mainline medicine and of the latter's allies in the sciences, industry, and government. As prods and gadflies, they not only keep America's tradition of medical diversity alive, but ensure that new or unpopular medical concepts continue to obtain at least some hearing and trial in American society. As such, they remain significant contributors to the processes of late-twentieth-century medical change and health improvement.

EPILOGUE

IF THERE is any single suitable descriptor for the American medical experience of the past four hundred years, it is its multifaceted and constantly shifting character. Several types of change have been highlighted or suggested in this book: the steadily shifting balance of medical influence and status among the large formative entities, or contributors to that experience; the changing health expectations of Americans in their various habitats; and the shifting of conflicting medical concepts and opposing health interests.

This book has given particular attention to the constantly changing roles of four entities that shaped America's medical world: orthodox medicine, nonestablishment medicine, science, and government. Throughout the colonial period, before there was a medical establishment, the dominant therapeutic force resided in the highly individualistic outlooks and unorganized activities of family and folk medical traditions. During the nineteenth century, under growing new pressures from mainline medicine, science, and government, these modes of therapy, along with traditional hygiene pursuits and the era's therapeutic sects, gradually declined in influence, at least among some segments of society. By 1900, in fact, most educated circles had dismissed such practices from consideration as serious elements of modern medicine. In the middle and late twentieth century, however, large numbers of Americans have been swept up in a new enthusiasm for hygienic ideals and regimens, while many others support alternative medical views and services, both on their own merits and as symbols of resistance to modern medical authority.

Orthodox medicine, by contrast, occupied a relatively insignificant place in the health thinking of Americans throughout the colonial period. Considerable numbers of practitioners began to associate themselves with mainline therapies and organizations in the late eighteenth century, with far more participating in the nineteenth century. They spent much of that period searching for professional identity and fighting for their lives economically against competing medical systems, however; substantial social influence and power thus eluded them throughout almost that entire span. Early in the twentieth century, regular medicine finally succeeded in overcoming much of the sectarian competition, gaining new public confidence, and assuming a position as the keystone of a formal medical establishment. Subsequently, until the 1990s, it has been vigorously consolidating and extending its power in the establishment by identifying closely with the methods and knowledge of modern laboratory science and by attempting to dominate the nation's health outlook and policies with its conservative agenda.

Another major entity, science, also had little immediate impact on seventeenth- and eighteenth-century medicine, except for that small number of well-to-do physicians or well-educated individuals who had the time and appetite for investigation. In the post-Revolutionary period science continued to lack relevance for the many physicians who thought of medicine as an art. Medical botany and climatology did flourish in the practical climate of early-nineteenth-century America, along with such medically related pursuits as phrenology and anthropology. But science began to assume a major role in the country's medicine only in the late nineteenth century, with the startlingly sudden and widespread realization of the importance of the laboratory and the adoption of its methods. In the twentieth century, the build-up and operation of the huge scientific establishment and spread of its research ethos has constituted a powerful and often overwhelming element in the century's medical life.

Governments, too, played limited medical roles during the colonial era, sharing their authority in this area with the church and deferring to traditional and individual practices except in dire emergencies. With the explosion of population in the hundred and fifty or so years following the American Revolution, governments at the various levels were reluctantly but steadily given additional health-related powers. On the one side, they came under ever more pressure to organize permanent measures against epidemic diseases as well as to make provisions for the health care of the destitute and other special groups. At the same time, the damaging conflicts of competing private medical interests and organizations increasingly forced governments to assume roles as arbitrators, regulators, and protectors of the public's health interests. By the mid-twentieth century, the federal government had thus assumed far-reaching influence over medical research and education, hospitals and health finance organizations, medications and foods, and other health matters. Not least, it financed and coordinated the country's many-sided efforts to combat diseases, though the emergence of new epidemics and epidemic conditions in every generation has tended to make for alarmingly elusive and shifting public health targets.

The country's manifold medical activities—orthodox, irregular, governmental, and scientific—were initiated and carried on over the years in direct or indirect response to a broad array of diseases, injuries, and other medical needs. Moreover, they were pursued in a context of natural and manmade environments and within a complex evolving framework of cultural, economic, social, and demographic circumstances, local and national. The sum total of these intersecting circumstances, settings, and activities has been considered in this book as America's basic health environment. But historically, the quality of this environment was far from uniform. It changed steadily from one generation to another. And, for citizens of every period, the health-related surroundings, resources, and expectations varied, sometimes drastically, depending on which of the nation's habitats they happened to be located in.

Colonial Era citizens in their small-town and rural habitats were often drastically affected healthwise by the harsh circumstances of their physical surroundings. Their health outlook was also deeply and inevitably colored by their destructive illnesses, impotent therapies, and short life expectancies. At the same time they were supported in these circumstances by the consolation of their religious faith as well as by the universally shared character of the centuries-old patterns of natural events—the repetitions of the seasons and agricultural practices; the successions of births, suffering, and death.

Nineteenth-century Americans were far less homogeneous than their ancestors in their habitats and thus in their expectations of health and health care. Those who joined the great migratory waves west and south or pursued transient lives for any considerable time seldom had access to any kind of medication or health care beyond what they provided for themselves. Those who stayed on the land as farmers or in small towns, in turn, retained much of the earlier patterns of low expectations, reconciliations, and limited benefit from medical, scientific, or governmental innovation. But those who moved into the cities often participated in those benefits, albeit in differing degrees. The urban well-to-do were increasingly able to take advantage of new therapeutic options, enjoyed higher standards of living and longer life expectancies, were provided with expanded sanitary services by governments, and were aware of new hopes offered by science. At the opposite end were city dwellers who could supply themselves only minimally with the necessities of life, were the most often exposed to dangerous diseases or accidents, were often left out of sanitary provisions made by governments, who had to make do with poorly informed healers and limited medications, and in serious illnesses were all too often subjected to degrading experiences in hospitals, almshouses, or other charities.

In the twentieth century the differentiations in America's health environments have been increasingly determined by economic factors. For the well-off populations of cities, small towns, and countryside alike, the range of health expectations and options have come to include the whole array of governmental public health and sanitary services, numerous hygienic activities and recreational facilities, the community's private and public health care institutions, personnel, and services, an enviable standard of living, and a life expectancy over twice that of the seventeenth century. The poor, wherever they live, have shared few of these expectations and have access to few of these health services. At the same time, for poor and well-to-do alike, the hygienic quality of life in nearly every habitat continues to decline in the wake of generations of uncontrolled urban development, heedless overexploitation of natural resources, and the gross pollution of environments by the products and toxic wastes of industry.

The American medical experience has thus included the opposing viewpoints, contrasting needs, and conflicting objectives of the populations of the various dissimilar habitats, as well as the often contradictory interests and opposing stakes of medicine's large contributory entities: governments, orthodox medicine, nonestablishment medicine, and science. Across time, medicine was constantly being altered by the struggles, compromises, and accommodations among partisans of the many conflicting views and interests. The peculiar medical character of every time period in American history is therefore sharply illuminated and pointed up for the historian by a variety of distinctive dichotomies and contrasts.

The seventeenth-century medical experience included, for instance, the abnormal mass mania and hysteria of the witchcraft episode, but it was even more deeply marked by the habitual fatalism of the colonists' normal confrontation with disease and death. Again, the initiative of prominent men in bringing European formal medical learning to America was clearly a significant aspect of that century's medical activity; but equally important and of far wider impact at the time was the practical nursing, birthing, gathering of herbs, and dosing done by women in the home.

For the eighteenth century, the continuing mixed character of medicine is illustrated in part by the image of the period's clergy as strong early supporters of inoculation, while the medical professions were long-time opponents of that measure. During the same period, the ferments of the Enlightenment opened up fresh new outlooks on philosophy and science for American intellectuals, but the ordinary man often continued to entertain older astrological and alchemical beliefs bearing on health.

In the nineteenth century, the contradictions and contrasts became more numerous. Selecting from among them, the historian is impressed by the image that has been passed down through time of Benjamin Rush as a kind of therapeutic monster because of the excesses of his heroic therapies; but this must be offset by the equally compelling picture of Rush the medical humanitarian. In that century the country also gained no little fame for its daring surgical operations, but the luster of those achievements is tarnished by a recollection of the age's badly mutilated patients. For the regular physician, the nineteenth century's significant medical contributions were typically those of an accumulation of pioneer medical heroes who were predominantly WASP, male, and aggressively orthodox in therapeutics. But the historian is quickly made aware that as the century went on a second American pantheon began to fill up, this one with pioneer medical heroes who were females, blacks, Catholics and Jews, and irregular practitioners ranging from botanics, hydropaths, and homeopaths to Christian Scientists and chiropractors.

The medical dichotomies of the twentieth century are no less striking or numerous. The medical character of the century is epitomized for many by the images of masked surgeons in hectic intensive care units and of white-coated scientists in the laboratories of vast and impersonal research centers; but offsetting these are images of socially involved nurses in other settings—at urban settlement houses, in rural Appalachia, and in quiet hospices. The century has been an age in which psychiatrists and others were prompt in devoting attention to the neuroses of the middle and upper classes, while governments, employers, unions, and epidemiologists alike have been slow in coming to grips with such deadly lower-class ailments as the black lung of the coal miners, the brown lung of the cotton-mill workers, and the pesticide poisoning of migrant workers. Finally, late-twentieth-century Americans are often impressed that their nation spends a larger proportion of its gross national product on health than any other developed country. But they are conspicuously slow in facing up to the fact that the general rate of infant mortality in the United States remains higher than that of all but a few other developed nations, and that it is twice as high for black infants as for white infants.

BIBLIOGRAPHICAL ESSAY

THIS ESSAY acknowledges monographic works that I found particularly helpful during the preparation of this book. It does not attempt to incorporate collateral works in general or social history, nor, regrettably, does it include journal articles, however valuable. It likewise omits all but a few of the relevant dissertations. However, the works that have been included will amplify in varying degrees the many matters that I have only been able to touch on lightly in my text. The works cited are diverse in viewpoint and uneven in quality. To note that there are still large gaps in their overall coverage of America's medical history is to state the obvious as well as to point to the needs and opportunities for further research in this field of scholarship.

General Works

The general history of medicine from early times, particularly in the "Western" context, is covered by a number of standard one-volume works. A balanced account is Charles J. Singer and E. A. Underwood, *A Short History of Medicine*, 2d ed. (1962). Fielding H. Garrison, *An Introduction to the History of Medicine*, 4th ed. (1929), is awkwardly organized but remains the most convenient source of much wanted information. Erwin H. Ackerknecht, *A Short History of Medicine*, rev. ed. (1968), is a highly concise interpretation, while Robert H. Hudson, *Disease and its Control: The Shaping of Modern Thought* (1983), is a competent recent study.

A number of works deal with European medicine during America's formative years. Outstanding in tracing the relationships between the two continents is Richard H. Shryock, *The Development of Modern Medicine: An Interpretation of the Social and Scientific Factors Involved*, enl. ed. (1947). The contributions in Allen G. Debus, ed.,

Medicine in Seventeenth Century England (1974), provide thorough coverage of learned medicine of that era, as does Lester S. King for the subsequent period, in his *The Medical World of the Eighteenth Century* (1958). Valuable studies of special aspects of medicine in the eighteenth and early nineteenth centuries include Erwin H. Ackerknecht, *Medicine at the Paris Hospital, 1794–1848* (1967); Michel Foucault, *The Birth of the Clinic* (1973); and Guenter B. Risse, *Hospital Life in Enlightenment Scotland: Care and Teaching at the Royal Infirmary of Edinburgh* (1986).

Assessments and critiques of modern medicine abound. Particularly provocative from the political and economic viewpoint is Ivan Illich, *Medical Nemesis: The Expropriation of Health* (1976); a forceful response to that work is David F. Horrobin, *Medical Hubris: A Reply to Ivan Illich* (1978). Another challenging study, particularly in its scientific analysis of historical data, is Thomas McKeown, *The Role of Medicine: Dream, Mirage or Nemesis?*, 2d ed. (1979). The collected essays in Asa Briggs and Julian H. Shelley, eds., *Science, Medicine and the Community: The Last Hundred Years* (1986), provide the combined insights of medical and other professionals. A similar work, but focusing upon the American medical scene, is John A. Knowles, ed., *Doing Better and Feeling Worse: Health in the United States* (1977).

The United States still lacks a definitive general study of its medical history. Pending such a work, an excellent introduction is provided by the short interpretive works of Richard H. Shryock, particularly his *Medicine and Society in America, 1660–1860* (1960); and his *Medicine in America: Historical Essays* (1966). These should be supplemented by James Bordley III and A. McGehee Harvey, *Two Centuries of American Medicine, 1776–1976* (1976), a highly detailed and useful work that is admittedly physician-oriented and whiggishly presentist in its focus. John Duffy, *The Healers: The Rise of the Medical Establishment* (1976), is an important survey from a broader historical viewpoint but one that gives insufficient attention to the twentieth century. By contrast, Paul Starr, *The Social Transformation of American Medicine* (1982), is most successful with the post–Civil War period, while John S. Haller, *American Medicine in Transition, 1840–1910* (1981), provides a useful bridge between the early and the modern periods. Whitfield J. Bell, Jr., *The Colonial Physician and Other Essays* (1975), is indispensable for the pre-1775 period. Maurice B. Gordon, *Aesculapius Comes to the Colonies* (1949), provides further detail on that period, while Ronald L. Numbers, ed., *Medicine in the New World: New Spain, New France, and New England* (1987), adds a valuable comparative context.

Collective works have become increasingly important in making available both original source materials and the recent scholarship of American medical history. For the former, a useful work is Gert H. Brieger, ed., *Medical America in the Nineteenth Century: Readings from the Literature* (1972); while Judith W. Leavitt and Ronald L. Numbers, eds., *Sickness and Health in America: Readings in the History of Medicine and Public Health*, 2d ed., rev. (1985), presents the reprinted articles of numerous historians. Susan Reverby and David Rosner, eds., *Health Care in America: Essays in Social History* (1979), and Morris J. Vogel and Charles E. Rosenberg, eds., *The Therapeutic Revolution: Essays in the Social History of American Medicine* (1979), are shorter but equally challenging collections. John Z. Bowers and Elizabeth F. Purcell, eds., *Advances in American Medicine: Essays at the Bicentennial*, 2 vols. (1976), is useful for its informed reviews of the recent history of the medical sciences by active participants in the various fields.

Regional histories of medicine are scarce and usually limited in scope. Richard Dunlop, *Doctors of the American Frontier* (1965), is one of the better older works. James O. Breeden, ed., *Medicine in the West* (1982), is informative but all too short. Southern medical history, on the other hand, is now exceptionally well served by two new collections of scholarly papers: Ronald L. Numbers and Todd L. Savitt, eds., *Science and Medicine in the Old South* (1989); and Todd L. Savitt and James Harvey Young, eds., *Disease and Distinctiveness in the American South* (1988).

State and local histories of medicine are numerous, but all too often they are both parochial and unscholarly. Models of what these works can be are David L. Cowen, *Medicine and Health in New Jersey: A History* (1964); and Thomas N. Bonner, *Medicine in Chicago* (1957). Also informative is Thomas N. Bonner, *The Kansas Doctor: A Century of Pioneering* (1959). Significant collective volumes are Philip Cash, Eric H. Christianson, and J. Worth Estes, eds., *Medicine in Colonial Massachusetts 1620–1820* (1980); and Ronald L. Numbers and Judith Walzer Leavitt, eds., *Wisconsin Medicine: Historical Perspectives* (1981). John Duffy, ed., *The Rudolph Matas History of Medicine in Louisiana*, 2 vols. (1958, 1962), is a solid longer contribution. Two other long works, Wyndham B. Blanton, *Medicine in Virginia*, 3 vols. (1930, 1931, 1933), and Joseph I. Waring, *A History of Medicine in South Carolina*, 3 vols. (1964, 1967, 1971), include much valuable detail but little interpretation.

Biographies and autobiographies abound of figures of varying importance in every aspect of America's medical history, though many are so hero-worshipping in character as to be of little value. Some of the more important and informative biographies will be referred to below under the special areas of medicine that their subjects influenced. In this section I include only a few that deal with particularly prominent individuals or illustrate some of the broader aspects of medical history. Whitfield J. Bell, Jr., *John Morgan, Continental Doctor* (1965), and Carl Binger, *Revolutionary Doctor: Benjamin Rush, 1746–1813* (1966), treat key characters at the beginning of formal medicine in America's Revolutionary age. Henry D. Shapiro and Zane L. Miller, eds., *Physician to the West: Selected Writings of Daniel Drake on Science and Society* (1970), while minimal in personal details, includes a wealth of information pertaining to nineteenth-century medical expansion in the Midwest. Eleanor M. Tilton, *Amiable Autocrat: A Biography of Dr. Oliver Wendell Holmes* (1947), is a highly readable treatment of a leader of mid-nineteenth-century Boston's medical elite, while Gerald N. Grob, *Edward Jarvis and the Medical World of Nineteenth-Century America* (1978), is a perceptive and valuable study. Considerable insight into antebellum southern medicine is afforded by James Breeden, *Joseph Jones, M.D.: Scientist of the Old South* (1975); and Reginald Horsman, *Josiah Nott of Mobile: Southerner, Physician, and Racial Theorist* (1987). Three splendid final biographies go far in providing an understanding of the coming of scientific medicine to this country: Simon Flexner and James T. Flexner, *William Henry Welch and the Heroic Age of American Medicine* (1941); Harvey Cushing, *The Life of Sir William Osler* (1948); and Donald Fleming, *William H. Welch and the Rise of Modern Medicine* (1987).

Diseases and Hospitals

There is no comprehensive history of the impact of disease in this country. However, John Duffy, *Epidemics in Colonial America* (1953), is an invaluable study of a particular period. Franklin H. Top, ed., *The History of American Epidemiology* (1952), is a useful account of official and scientific concerns for the infectious diseases.

The American experience with many of the major individual disease conditions has been extensively written about, though large gaps remain. Among the epidemic diseases, a cameo study of diphtheria is Ernest Caulfield, *A True History of the Terrible Epidemic Vulgarly Called the Throat Distemper which Occurred in His Majesty's New England Colonies Between the Years 1735 and 1740* (1934). The partly autobiographical work, Hans Zinsser, *Rats, Lice, and History*, 4th ed. (1942), is a classic study of typhus. The history of yellow fever may be approached through Howard A. Kelly, *Walter Reed and Yellow Fever*, 3d ed. (1906); John Duffy, *Sword of Pestilence: The New Orleans Yellow Fever Epidemic of 1853* (1966); and the evocative work by John

H. Powell, *Bring Out Your Dead: The Great Plague of Yellow Fever in Philadelphia in 1793* (1949). Charles E. Rosenberg, *The Cholera Years: The United States in 1832, 1849, and 1866*, new ed. (1987), has set the standard for social histories of diseases. The influenza pandemic of 1918 is excellently handled in Alfred W. Crosby, *Epidemic and Peace, 1918* (1976). And the scientific aspects of modern polio are thoroughly presented in John R. Paul, *A History of Poliomyelitis* (1971); and Saul Benison, *Tom Rivers; Reflections on a Life in Medicine and Science: An Oral History* (1967).

The history of endemic disease conditions has been receiving increased attention. Among the best treatments of malaria are St. Julien Ravenel Childs, *Malaria and Colonization in the Carolina Low Country, 1526–1696* (1940); and Erwin H. Ackerknecht, *Malaria in the Upper Mississippi Valley 1760–1900* (1945). Milton Terris, ed., *Goldberger on Pellagra* (1964), and Elizabeth W. Etheridge, *The Butterfly Caste: A Social History of Pellagra in the South* (1972), provide valuable complementary treatments of this diet-deficiency disease. For hookworm disease, John Ettling, *The Germ of Laziness: Rockefeller Philanthropy and Public Health in the New South* (1981), is a particularly penetrating interpretation. The scientific history of tuberculosis has been examined by Selman A. Waksman, *The Conquest of Tuberculosis* (1964), while that disease's social and institutional aspects are stressed in Robert Taylor, *Saranac: America's Magic Mountain* (1986); and Mark Caldwell, *The Last Crusade: The War on Consumption, 1862–1954* (1988). Richard H. Shryock, *National Tuberculosis Association, 1904–1954* (1957), ably reviews the early decades of one of the largest of the voluntary health organizations. Major studies of two diseases that were long unmentionable in polite society are Allan M. Brandt, *No Magic Bullet: A Social History of Venereal Disease in the United States Since 1880, With a New Chapter on AIDS* (1987); and James T. Patterson, *The Dread Disease: Cancer and Modern American Culture* (1987).

For drug addiction, see the following perceptive and complementary works: David F. Musto, *The American Disease: Origins of Narcotic Control*, new ed. (1987); H. Wayne Morgan, *Drugs in America: A Social History 1800–1980* (1981); and David T. Courtwright, *Dark Paradise: Opium Addiction in America before 1940* (1982). Nineteenth-century drinking habits and alcoholism are solidly treated in W. J. Rorabaugh, *The Alcoholic Republic: An American Tradition* (1979); and Ian R. Tyrrell, *Sobering Up: From Temperance to Prohibition in Antebellum America, 1800–1860* (1979).

Competent general histories of mental disease include Albert Deutsch, *The Mentally Ill in America* (1949); and Norman Dain, *Concepts of Insanity in the United States, 1789–1865* (1964). For the early-twentieth-century mental hygiene movement, see Clifford W. Beers, *A Mind That Found Itself*, 7th ed. (1948); and Barbara Sicherman, "The Quest for Mental Health in America, 1880–1917," Ph.D. diss. (1967). Harold Schwartz, *Samuel Gridley Howe, Social Reformer, 1801–1876* (1956), examines New England's concerns for mental disease, mental retardation, and the blind in a broad social and political context.

While accounts of individual hospitals have been numerous throughout this century, serious historical attention to the hospital as a social and scientific institution has been lacking until very recently. A relatively early exception is Leonard K. Eaton, *New England Hospitals, 1790–1833* (1957). Charles Rosenberg, *The Care of Strangers: The Rise of America's Hospital System* (1987) has now provided a highly substantial and insightful study of hospitals up to the 1920s. This work has been extended timewise, particularly in its economic and organizational aspects, by the equally meritorious study by Rosemary Stevens, *In Sickness and in Wealth: American Hospitals in the Twentieth Century* (1989). Two fine works deal with the transformation of hospital care in particular late-nineteenth-century and early-twentieth-century communities: Morris J. Vogel, *The Invention of the Modern Hospital: Boston 1870–1930* (1980); and David Rosner, *A Once Charitable Enterprise: Hospitals and Health Care in Brooklyn and New York, 1885–1915* (1982). For municipal institutions, see Harry Dowling, *City Hospitals: The Undercare of the Underprivileged* (1982). The exceptional role that one hospital and its affiliated medical school has played in modern scientific medicine is recounted in Alan M. Chesney, *The Johns Hopkins Hospital and the Johns Hopkins University School of Medicine: A Chronicle*, 3 vols. (1943–1963).

The historiography of America's mental institutions was long virtually limited to Helen F. Marshall, *Dorothea Dix, Forgotten Samaritan* (1937). The recent awakening of further scholarly interest in such hospitals owes much to David J. Rothman, *The Discovery of the Asylum: Social Order and Disorder in the New Republic* (1971). For a comprehensive treatment of the subject, however, see Gerald N. Grob, *Mental Institutions in America: Social Policy to 1875* (1973); and his sequel, *Mental Illness and American Society, 1875–1940* (1983).

Mainline Medicine and Professions

The general development of professionalism has been examined in several good studies. The early traumas of this development are ably discussed in Henry B. Shafer, *The American Medical Profession, 1783–1850* (1936); Joseph F. Kett, *The Formation of the American Medical Pro-*

fession: The Role of Institutions 1780–1860 (1980); and William G. Rothstein, *American Physicians in the Nineteenth Century* (1972). For more recent aspects, see James G. Burrow, *Organized Medicine in the Progressive Era: The Move to Monopoly* (1977); and Bernard J. Stern, *American Medical Practices in the Perspective of a Century* (1945). Barbara Ehrenreich and John Ehrenreich, *The American Health Empire: Power, Profits, and Politics* (1970), presents a radical viewpoint. Jeffrey L. Berlant, *Profession and Monopoly: A Study of Medicine in the United States and Great Britain* (1975), is a useful comparative work.

For the American Medical Association, James G. Burrow, *AMA: Voice of American Medicine* (1963) provides a historian's perspective. Morris Fishbein et al., *A History of the American Medical Association, 1847 to 1947* (1947), is written by physicians. Another important national medical society is reviewed in A. McGehee Harvey, *The Association of American Physicians 1886–1986: A Century of Progress in Medical Science* (1986). The careers of two particularly influential medical journalists are examined in Courtney Robert Hall, *A Scientist in the Early Republic: Samuel Latham Mitchill, 1764–1831* (1934); and Morris Fishbein, *Morris Fishbein, M.D.: An Autobiography* (1969).

Details of the physician's practice have been examined from several sides. Efforts at internal and public regulation of physicians have been summarized in Richard H. Shryock, *Medical Licensing in America, 1650–1965* (1967). The profession's early attempt to standardize "doctor bills" is discussed in George Rosen, *Fees and Fee Bills: Some Economic Aspects of Medical Practice in Nineteenth-Century America* (1946). John Harley Warner, *The Therapeutic Perspective: Medical Practice, Knowledge and Identity in America, 1820–1885* (1986), is a rich and highly original analysis of changing modes of healing. Steps taken to regulate the individual physician's relations to his profession and to society are discussed in Donald E. Konold, *A History of American Medical Ethics, 1847–1912* (1962); and Chester R. Burns, "Medical Ethics in the United States Before the Civil War," Ph.D. diss. (1969). The definitive studies of medical quackery are James Harvey Young, *The Toadstool Millionaires: A Social History of Patent Medicines in America before Federal Regulation* (1961); and his *The Medical Messiahs: A Social History of Health Quackery in Twentieth-Century America* (1967).

The training of physicians has been discussed comprehensively in Kenneth M. Ludmerer, *Learning to Heal: The Development of American Medical Education* (1985). A short text is Martin Kaufman, *American Medical Education: The Formative Years 1765–1910* (1976). William P. Norwood, *Medical Education in the United States before the Civil War* (1944), focuses on the organization of early medical schools. Ronald L. Numbers, ed., *The Education of American Physicians* (1980), examines the development of education in the various medical specialties and allied professions. Thomas Bonner, *American Doctors and German Universities, 1870–1914* (1963), is an invaluable study of professional and scientific study abroad. William G. Rothstein, *American Medical Schools and the Practice of Medicine: A History* (1987), is a timely if uneven interpretation of the effects of modern medical science and specialization on the teaching function of medical schools.

General aspects of the development of medical specialization have been admirably covered by Rosemary Stevens, *American Medicine and the Public Interest* (1971). Most of the individual specialties, however, still await careful historical examination. Among the exceptions, for the general history of surgery, see Allen O. Whipple, *The Evolution of Surgery in the United States* (1963), but a more socially oriented study is needed. Frederick F. Cartwright, *The Development of Modern Surgery* (1968), considers post-1800 American contributors in the context of their European contemporaries. Among the most useful biographies of modern surgeons, see John F. Fulton, *Harvey Cushing, a Biography* (1946); and Peter C. English, *Shock, Physiological Surgery and George Washington Crile: Medical Innovation in the Progressive Era* (1980). Martin S. Pernick, *A Calculus of Suffering: Pain, Professionalism and Anesthesia in Nineteenth-Century America* (1985), is an original and sensitive account of social discrimination in early surgical intervention.

Two significant large histories of childbirth and obstetrics in this country are Judith Waltzer Leavitt, *Brought to Bed: Childbearing in America 1750 to 1950* (1986); and Richard W. Wertz and Dorothy C. Wertz, *Lying-In: A History of Childbirth in America*, enl. ed. (1989). Both, among other matters, highlight the growing tensions between women and the modern medical care establishment over control of childbirth. A shorter work is Judy B. Litoff, *American Midwives: 1860 to the Present* (1978). For the professional development of pediatrics, see Thomas E. Cone, Jr., *History of American Pediatrics* (1979).

The early history of psychiatry is dealt with in American Psychiatric Association, ed., *One Hundred Years of American Psychiatry* (1944); and Ruth B. Caplan, *Psychiatry and the Community in Nineteenth-Century America* (1969). But see also the works by Grob, Dain, and others listed earlier under Diseases and Hospitals. The impact of Freud in this country has been thoroughly examined in John C. Burnham, *Psychoanalysis in American Medicine, 1894–1918: Medicine, Science, and Culture* (1967); and Nathan G. Hale, *Freud and the Americans: The Beginnings of Psychoanalysis in the United States, 1876–1917* (1971).

Among the health professions associated with medicine, nursing has been one of the most adequately treated, historically. An early work, Richard H. Shryock, *The History of Nursing* (1959), places American nursing in a context of foreign developments. Philip A. Kalisch and Beatrice Kalisch, *The Advance of American Nursing* (1978), is a useful text. One of nursing's specialties is examined in Karen Buhler-Wilkerson, "False Dawn: The Rise and Decline of Public Health Nursing, 1900–1930," Ph.D. diss. (1984). Valuable recent interpretations are Barbara Melosh, *"The Physician's Hand": Work, Culture and Conflict in American Nursing* (1982); and Susan Reverby, *Ordered to Care: The Dilemma of American Nursing, 1850–1945* (1987).

For the profession of pharmacy, the best general account of American developments is to be found in Glenn Sonnedecker, *Kremers and Urdang's History of Pharmacy*, 4th ed. (1976). The only extensive history of veterinary medicine is J. F. Smithcors, *The American Veterinary Profession: Its Background and Development* (1963), a work which, though poorly organized, is filled with useful detail. American dentistry also has no adequate general history. However, see Robert W. McCluggage, *A History of the American Dental Association: A Century of Health Service* (1959); and Ruth Roy Harris, *Dental Science in a New Age: A History of the National Institute of Dental Research* (1989).

Lay Health Activities and Alternative Medicine

There is much room for further historical work in these areas. The widest-ranging scholarly treatments of such topics to date are Norman Gevitz, ed., *Other Healers: Unorthodox Medicine in America* (1988); and William B. Walker, "The Health Reform Movement in the United States, 1830–1870," Ph.D. diss. (1955).

Among special studies pertaining to the personal pursuit of health, a valuable compendium is Wayland D. Hand, ed., *American Folk Medicine: A Symposium* (1973). Guenter B. Risse, Ronald L. Numbers, and Judith W. Leavitt, eds., *Medicine without Doctors: Home Health Care in American History* (1977), examines health expedients beyond the level of folk remedies. Stephen W. Nissenbaum, *Sex, Diet, and Debility in Jacksonian America: Sylvester Graham and Health Reform* (1980), and Richard W. Schwartz, *John Henry Kellogg, M.D.* (1970), are useful studies of central figures in nineteenth-century hygiene causes. Medical travel to spas and health resorts is dealt with in Billy M. Jones, *Health-Seekers in the Southwest, 1817–1900* (1967). Martha H. Verbrugge, *Able-Bodied Womanhood: Personal Health and Social Change in Nineteenth-Century Boston* (1988), competently examines health reform in the light of women's needs and aspirations.

Americans' concern for diet is an important part of the Nissenbaum and Schwartz works cited above. Richard O. Cummings, *The*

American and His Food, rev. ed. (1941), a broader review of food habits and nutrition, is still useful. But see also Harvey Levenstein, *Revolution at the Table: The Transformation of the American Diet* (1988). Biographies of significant innovators in nutrition and home economics include Caroline L. Hunt, *The Life of Ellen H. Richards* (1912); and Emma Seifrit Weigley, *Sarah Tyson Rorer: The Nation's Instructress in Dietetics and Cookery* (1977). The history of exercise and physical improvement is well covered in James C. Whorton, *Crusaders for Fitness: The History of American Health Reformers* (1982); and Harvey Green, *Fit for America: Health Fitness, Sport, and American Society* (1986). Further details are presented in Earle Ziegler, ed., *A History of Physical Education and Sport in the United States and Canada* (1975).

Several of the principal therapeutic sects have individual histories. Homeopathy is sympathetically and thoroughly treated by Harris L. Coulter, *Science and Ethics in American Medicine, 1800–1914* (1973); more traditionally (skeptically) and concisely in Martin Kaufman, *Homeopathy in America: The Rise and Fall of a Medical Heresy* (1971). John D. Davies, *Phrenology, Fad and Science: A Nineteenth-Century American Crusade* (1955), is a competent account. Madeleine B. Stern, *Heads and Headlines: The Phrenological Fowlers* (1971), is a historical gem dealing with several of the mid-nineteenth-century leaders of health reform. Hydropathy is covered interestingly in Harry B. Weiss and Howard R. Kemble, *The Great American Water-Cure Craze: A History of Hydropathy in the United States* (1967); and in more scholarly form in Jane B. Donegan, *Hydropathic Highway to Health: Women and Water-Cure in Antebellum America* (1986). Norman Gevitz, *The D.O.'s: Osteopathic Medicine in America* (1982), is an able and balanced work.

Religious healers and therapeutic movements are considered in several works. For the early period, see Patricia Ann Watson, "The Angelical Conjunction: The Preacher-Physicians of Colonial New England," Ph.D. diss. (1987). An important study of one such preacher is Otto T. Beall, Jr. and Richard H. Shryock, *Cotton Mather: First Significant Figure in American Medicine* (1954). Another biography, Ronald L. Numbers, *Prophetess of Health: A Study of Ellen G. White* (1976), provides a balanced examination of the hygienic precepts of the founder of Seventh-Day Adventism. Herbert G. Jackson, *The Spirit Rappers* (1972), discusses nineteenth-century spiritualism. Christian Science and other mental healing movements are dealt with in Raymond J. Cunningham, "Ministry of Healing: The Origins of the Psychotherapeutic Role of the American Churches," Ph.D. diss. (1965). David E. Harrell, Jr., *All Things Are Possible: The Healing and Charismatic Revivals in Modern America* (1975), is a useful survey.

Science and Research

While there is still no single comprehensive work on the history of American science, a convenient introduction is George H. Daniels, *Science in American Society: A Social History* (1971). Among a number of works that examine particular periods, especially important are: Raymond Phineas Stearns, *Science in the British Colonies of America* (1970); Brooke Hindle, *The Pursuit of Science in Revolutionary America* (1956); John C. Greene, *American Science in the Age of Jefferson* (1984); George H. Daniels, *American Science in the Age of Jackson* (1968); and Robert V. Bruce, *The Launching of Modern American Science, 1846–1876* (1987). A perceptive and useful regional history is Dirk Jan Struik, *Yankee Science in the Making*, rev. ed. (1962). Informative studies of the sources of support for science are Howard S. Miller, *Dollars for Research: Science and its Patrons in Nineteenth-Century America* (1970); and Eli Ginzberg and Anna B. Dutka, *The Financing of Biomedical Research* (1989). Two large works are devoted to the significant roles played by scientific societies: Alexandra Oleson and Sanborn C. Brown, eds., *The Pursuit of Knowledge in the Early American Republic: American Scientific and Learned Societies from Colonial Times to the Civil War* (1976); and their *The Organization of Knowledge in Modern America, 1860–1920* (1979). A. Hunter Dupree, *Science in the Federal Government: A History of Policies and Activities to 1940* (1957), is invaluable. Recent developments in sciences impinging closely upon medicine are dealt with in Robert E. Kohler, *From Medical Chemistry to Biochemistry: The Making of a Biomedical Discipline* (1982); and Garland E. Allen, *Life Science in the Twentieth Century* (1975), both of them indispensable studies.

A knowledgeable, though by now partly outdated, overview of the medical sciences in this country is Richard H. Shryock, *American Medical Research Past and Present* (1947). A more recent view is A. McGehee Harvey, *Science at the Bedside: Clinical Research in American Medicine, 1905–1945* (1981). Important special studies are Stanley G. Reiser, *Medicine and the Reign of Technology* (1978); and Audrey P. Davis, *Medicine and Its Technology: An Introduction to the History of Medical Instrumentation* (1978). Research activities and support programs of the National Institutes of Health are well treated in Victoria A. Harden, *Inventing the NIH: Federal Biomedical Research Policy, 1887–1937* (1986); and Stephen P. Strickland, *Politics, Science and Dread Disease* (1972); together with Strickland's *The Story of the NIH Grants Programs* (1988). The first half-century of one of America's most important early biomedical research centers is ably surveyed in George

W. Corner, *A History of the Rockefeller Institute, 1901–1953* (1964). For animal research and the antivivisection movement, see the sensitive works of James Turner, *Reckoning with the Beast: Animals, Pain and Humanity in the Victorian Mind* (1980); and Susan M. Lederer, "Human Experimentation and Antivivisection in Turn-of-the-Century America," Ph.D. diss. (1987).

The individual medical sciences differ noticeably in the historical treatment they have received. Physiology has been particularly well covered by such recent works as Gerald L. Geison, ed., *Physiology in the American Context, 1850–1940* (1987); Saul Benison, A. Clifford Barger, and Elin H. Wolfe, *Walter B. Cannon: The Life and Times of a Young Scientist* (1987); and Bruce Fye, *The Development of American Physiology: Scientific Medicine in the Nineteenth Century* (1987). Esmond R. Long, *A History of American Pathology* (1962), is a standard reference tool, while careers of bacteriologists and related scientists are conveniently summarized in Paul F. Clark, *Pioneer Microbiologists of America* (1961). For botany, an introductory work is Joseph A. Ewan, ed., *A Short History of Botany in the United States* (1969); while the botanical interests of early physicians are the focus of Dorothy I. Lansing, ed., *Medicine and Science in Early America: Being the Collected Essays of George Edmund Gifford, Jr.* (1982). Two works bearing upon medical anthropology and racial theories are the excellent volume of William Stanton, *The Leopard's Spots: Scientific Attitudes toward Race in America 1815–1859* (1960); and an important complementary study, John S. Haller, Jr., *Outcasts from Evolution: Scientific Attitudes of Racial Inferiority, 1859–1900* (1971).

For psychology, there is a need for an up-to-date general and social history. Splendid biographies of two major early figures in the field are Ralph Barton Perry, *The Thought and Character of William James*, 2 vols. (1935); and Dorothy Ross, *G. Stanley Hall: The Psychologist as Prophet* (1972). A meaty and valuable examination of the field's technical side is Michael M. Sokal, ed., *Psychological Testing and American Society, 1890–1930* (1987). The early history of quantification in American medicine and society is covered in Patricia Cline Cohen, *A Calculating People: The Spread of Numeracy in Early America* (1982); and James H. Cassedy, *American Medicine and Statistical Thinking, 1800–1860* (1984).

The scientific aspects of modern pharmaceutical manufacturing are competently dealt with in Jonathan Liebenau, *Medical Science and Medical Industry: The Formation of the American Pharmaceutical Industry* (1987); and John P. Swann, *Academic Scientists and the Pharmaceutical Industry: Cooperative Research in Twentieth-Century America* (1988). For genetics, particular attention has been given to the eugenics movement. Among the most useful works, see Mark H. Haller, *Eugenics: Hereditarian Attitudes in American Thought* (1963); Kenneth M. Ludmerer, *Genetics and American Society: A Historical Appraisal* (1972); and Daniel J. Kevles, *In the Name of Eugenics: Genetics and the Uses of Human Heredity* (1985). A biographical study of a major geneticist is Garland E. Allen, *Thomas Hunt Morgan: The Man and His Science* (1976).

Social Aspects of Health and Medicine

Several solid studies explore the historical incidence of poverty in this country and community efforts to relieve it. Social perspectives on the problem are sensitively examined in Robert H. Bremner, *From the Depths: The Discovery of Poverty* (1956). Samuel Mencher, *Poor Law to Poverty Program: Economic Security Policy in Britain and the United States* (1967); Walter Trattner, *From Poor Law to Welfare State: A History of Social Welfare in America* (1974); and James Leiby, *A History of Social Welfare and Social Work in the United States* (1978), are important accounts of both private and governmental initiatives. For professional aspects, see Roy Lubove, *The Professional Altruist: The Emergence of Social Work as a Career, 1880–1930* (1965). Classic accounts of activities at urban settlement houses include Jane Addams, *Twenty Years at Hull House, with Autobiographical Notes* (1923); and Lillian D. Wald, *The House on Henry Street* (1915).

Broad reviews of private philanthropy over the years are Robert H. Bremner, *American Philanthropy* (1960); and Merle Curti, *American Philanthropy Abroad: A History* (1963). Excellent general histories of private foundations and their work include Warren Weaver, *U.S. Philanthropic Foundations—Their History, Structure, Management, and Record* (1967); and Ellen C. Lagemann, *Private Power for the Public Good: A History of the Carnegie Foundation for the Advancement of Teaching* (1983).

Standard histories of other foundations that have contributed heavily to medical pursuits include A. McGehee Harvey and Susan Abrams, *For the Welfare of Mankind: The Commonwealth Fund and American Medicine* (1986); and Raymond Fosdick, *The Story of the Rockefeller Foundation* (1952). Greer Williams, *The Plague Killers* (1969), deals with foreign programs of the Rockefeller philanthropies. E. Richard Brown, *Rockefeller Medicine Men: Medicine and Capitalism in America* (1979); and Howard S. Berliner, *A System of Scientific Medicine: Philanthropic Foundations in the Flexner Era* (1985) are Marxist interpretations. Foster Rhea Dulles, *The American Red Cross: A History* (1950), is a solid study of this important body and its work, but it needs updating.

The broad phases of America's demographic history are clearly presented in Robert V. Wells, *Revolutions in Americans' Lives: A Demographic Perspective on the History of Americans, Their Families, and Their Society* (1982). For population history, see W. S. Rossiter, *A Century of Population Growth* (1909); and Margo J. Anderson, *The American Census: A Social History* (1988). Studies of immigration include Oscar Handlin, ed., *Immigration as a Factor in American History* (1959); Maldwyn Allen Jones, *American Immigration* (1960); and David Ward, *Cities and Immigrants: A Century of Change in Nineteenth-Century America* (1971). The early relationships of medicine and demographic matters are examined in James H. Cassedy, *Demography in Early America: Beginnings of the Statistical Mind 1600–1800* (1969); and in his *Medicine and American Growth, 1800–1860* (1986).

Two valuable histories of American efforts to limit population include Linda Gordon, *Woman's Body, Woman's Right: A Social History of Birth Control in America* (1976), from the feminist viewpoint; and James Reed, *From Private Vice to Public Virtue: The Birth Control Movement and American Society since 1830* (1978), a more dispassionate treatment. For an able view of the principal early-twentieth-century leader of the movement, see David M. Kennedy, *Birth Control in America: The Career of Margaret Sanger* (1970). The early legal and social history of abortion is excellently presented in James C. Mohr, *Abortion in America: The Origins and Evolution of National Policy, 1800–1900* (1978). Useful examinations of early sexuality include John S. Haller and Robin M. Haller, *The Physician and Sexuality in Victorian America* (1974); and G. J. Barker-Benfield, *The Horrors of the Half-Known Life: Male Attitudes toward Women and Sexuality in Nineteenth-Century America* (1976).

Most of America's principal population segments have had their health problems and historical involvements in medicine examined to at least some extent. For the Indians, the devastating toll of disease resulting from their contacts with Europeans is persuasively dealt with in Alfred W. Crosby, *The Columbian Exchange: Biological and Cultural Consequences of 1492* (1972); in his *Ecological Imperialism: The Biological Expansion of Europe, 900–1900* (1986); and in Russell Thornton, *American Indian Holocaust and Survival: A Population History since 1492* (1987). An influential earlier work is E. Wagner Stearn and Allen E. Stearn, *The Effect of Smallpox on the Destiny of the Amerindian* (1945). Grant Foreman, *Indian Removal: The Emigration of the Five Civilized Tribes of Indians* (1932), takes into account the sickness and death that accompanied the Indian removals. Indigenous remedies and therapies practiced by the various tribal groups are summarized in Virgil J. Vogel, *American Indian Medicine* (1970). A frustratingly brief introduction to federal medical assistance to Indians is Ruth M. Raup, *The Indian Health Program from 1800 to 1955* (1959). For blacks, Philip D. Curtin, *The Atlantic Slave Trade: A Census* (1969), includes estimates of mortality occurring on the passage from Africa. Two useful works examine the health of blacks under slavery: William Dosite Postell, *The Health of Slaves of Southern Plantations* (1951); and Todd L. Savitt, *Medicine and Slavery: The Diseases and Health Care of Blacks in Antebellum Virginia* (1978). The hygienic plight of the freedmen is examined in J. Thomas May, "The Medical Care of Blacks in Louisiana during Occupation and Reconstruction, 1862–1868: Its Social and Political Background," Ph.D. diss. (1970). Special insight into the diseases of slaves is afforded by Kenneth F. Kiple and Virginia H. King, *Another Dimension to the Black Diaspora: Diet, Disease, and Racism* (1981). Blacks as physicians have been most broadly treated by Herbert Morais, *History of the Negro in Medicine* (1967). Special studies on recent phases of this same topic include Vanessa N. Gamble, ed., *Germs Have No Color Lines: Blacks and American Medicine, 1900–1945* (1988); and Claude H. Organ and Margaret M. Kosiba, eds., *A Century of Black Surgeons: The U.S.A. Experience* (1987).

The role of women in medicine has been competently examined by Mary Roth Walsh, *"Doctors Wanted: No Women Need Apply": Sexual Barriers in the Medical Profession, 1835–1975* (1977); and Regina Markell Morantz-Sanchez, *Sympathy and Science: Women Physicians in American Medicine* (1985). Elizabeth Blackwell, *Pioneer Work in Opening the Medical Profession to Women: Autobiographical Sketches*, rep. ed. (1977), is the life of one of the mid-nineteenth-century pathfinders. Margaret Rossiter, *Women Scientists in America: Struggles and Strategies* (1982), includes much on the various health sciences. Judith Waltzer Leavitt, ed., *Women and Health in America: Historical Readings* (1984), is a valuable anthology of studies on women in medicine and on women's diseases. Of special interest is Sarah Stage, *Female Complaints: Lydia Pinkham and the Business of Women's Medicine* (1979). Other aspects of women's health are discussed in Ronald G. Walters, *Primers for Prudery: Sexual Advice of Victorian America* (1974); and Barbara Ehrenreich and Deidre English, *For Her Own Good: 150 Years of the Experts' Advice to Women* (1978).

The beginnings of organized child health care are recalled in the autobiography of Sara Josephine Baker, *Fighting for Life* (1939). Histories of the United States Children's Bureau include D. E. Bradbury, *Four Decades of Action for Children: A Short History of the Children's Bureau* (1956); and Manfred J. Waserman, "The Emergence of Modern Child Health Care: Pediatrics, Public Health, and the Federal Government," Ph.D. diss. (1981). An intimate account of one of the Bureau's early leaders is Jane Addams, *My Friend, Julia Lathrop* (1935). One of the Bureau's important concerns is dealt with in Walter I. Trattner, *Crusade for the Children: A History of the National Child Labor Committee and Child Labor Reform in America* (1970). Two works deal with infant feeding: Thomas E. Cone, Jr., *200 Years of Feeding Infants in America* (1976); and Rima D. Apple, *Mothers and Medicine: A Social History of Infant Feeding, 1890–1950* (1987).

Historical insight into old age in this country is afforded by the diverse approaches of David Hackett Fisher, *Growing Old in America* (1977); W. Andrew Achenbaum, *Old Age in the New Land: The American Experience since 1790* (1978); and Carole Haber, *Beyond Sixty-Five: The Dilemma of Old Age in America's Past* (1983).

Public Health

There is no history of public health that covers its larger environmental and social ramifications as well as its professional elements. For a general review of Americans' relations with and attitudes toward the physical environment, see Roderick Nash, ed., *The American Environment: Readings in the History of Conservation* (1968). A unique exploration of the symbiotic relationships of human diseases in a regional environment is Albert Cowdrey, *This Land, This South: An Environmental History* (1983). General urban histories that place health matters in a context of the city's other problems include Charles N. Glaab and A. Theodore Brown, *A History of Urban America* (1967); and Sam Bass Warner, Jr., *The Urban Wilderness: A History of the American City* (1972). Mel Scott, *American City Planning since 1890* (1969), considers the roles of professional urban planners in the effort to improve the quality of life, while Samuel P. Hays, *Beauty, Health, and Permanence: Environmental Politics in the United States, 1955–1985* (1987), emphasizes the recent growth of such values among the general public.

Two useful general works on the history of environmental sanitation are Victoria V. Ozonoff, "Medicine, Social Reform, and the Built Environment," Ph.D. diss. (1984); and Martin V. Melosi, ed., *Pollution and Reform in American Cities, 1870–1930* (1980). Able studies of individual sanitary problems and reforms include Nelson Blake, *Water for the Cities* (1956); Roy Lubove, *The Progressives and the Slums: Tenement House Reform in New York, 1890–1917* (1962); and Martin V. Melosi, *Garbage in the Cities: Refuse, Reform, and the Environment, 1880–1980* (1981). James J. Farrell, *Inventing the American Way of Death, 1830–1920* (1980), examines mortuary and burial practices.

Occupational health and industrial medicine are covered broadly in Henry B. Selleck and Alfred H. Whittaker, *Occupational Health in America* (1962); Daniel M. Berman, *Death on the Job: Occupational Health and Safety Struggles in the United States* (1978); and David Rosner and Gerald Markowitz, eds., *Dying for Work: Workers' Safety and Health in Twentieth-Century America* (1989). A fine regional study is Edward H. Beardsley, *A History of Neglect: Health Care for Blacks and Mill Workers in the Twentieth-Century South* (1987). Barbara Sicherman, *Alice Hamilton: A Life in Letters* (1984), is an essential study of this early-twentieth-century pioneer of industrial medicine.

The best general history of public health in its professional and institutional aspects is John Duffy, *The Sanitarians: A History of American Public Health* (1990). Older histories that continue to be useful include Mazyck P. Ravenel, ed., *A Half-Century of Public Health* (1921); Wilson G. Smillie, *Public Health, Its Promise for the Future* (1955); and George Rosen, *Preventive Medicine in the United States 1900–1975: Trends and Interpretations* (1975).

Several substantial local public health histories are available. For the states, these include the pioneering work by Philip D. Jordan, *The Peoples' Health: A History of Public Health in Minnesota to 1948* (1953); and the more sophisticated study of Barbara Gutmann Rosenkrantz, *Public Health and the State: Changing Views in Massachusetts, 1842–1936* (1972). Particularly valuable works for individual cities are John B. Blake, *Public Health in the Town of Boston, 1630–1822* (1959); Judith Waltzer Leavitt, *The Healthiest City: Milwaukee and the Politics of Health Reform* (1982); the two volumes by Stuart Galishof, *Safeguarding the Public Health: Newark, 1895–1918* (1975), and his *Newark: The Nation's Unhealthiest City, 1832–1895* (1988); and the two-volume history by John Duffy, *A History of Public Health in New York City* (1968, 1974). Further details of public health developments in both the city and state of New York are found in the rich biography, Charles-Edward A. Winslow, *The Life of Hermann M. Biggs* (1929).

A study of one of the early scientific aspects of public health is John B. Blake, *Benjamin Waterhouse and the Introduction of Vaccination: A Reappraisal* (1957). Wade H. Oliver, *The Man Who Lived for Tomorrow* (1941), examines the life of William H. Park, long-time head of New York City's pioneering public health laboratory. James H. Cassedy, *Charles V. Chapin and the Public Health Movement* (1962), discusses the scientifically-based "new public health" of the early twentieth century. Harry Dowling, *Fighting Infection: Conquests of the Twentieth Century* (1977), is a useful review of the role of modern immunology and chemotherapy in the control of communicable disease.

Oscar E. Anderson, *The Health of a Nation* (1958) is a study of Harvey Wiley, the leader of food and drug reform in the early twentieth century. Later phases of that reform are considered in Charles O. Jackson, *Food and Drug Legislation in the New Deal* (1970); and James Whorton, *Before Silent Spring: Pesticides and Public Health in Pre-DDT America* (1974). The training of public health professionals is solidly presented in Elizabeth Fee, *Disease and Discovery: A History of the Johns Hopkins School of Hygiene and Public Health, 1916–1939* (1987). E. O. Jordan, G. C. Whipple, and C-E. A. Winslow, *A Pioneer of Public Health: William Thompson Sedgwick* (1924), while short and out of date, remains the only monographic account of the significant earlier educational programs in sanitation and public health at MIT and Harvard.

Political and Economic Factors: Federal Health Pursuits

General studies of the political and economic aspects of medicine include Odin W. Anderson, *Health Services in the United States: A Growth Enterprise since 1875* (1985); and Lloyd C. Taylor, *The Medical Profession and Social Reform, 1885–1945* (1974). A thoughtful comparative work is Daniel M. Fox, *Health Policies, Health Politics: The British and American Experience, 1911–1965* (1986). Particular economic matters are dealt with in Odin W. Anderson, *The Uneasy Equilibrium: Private and Public Financing of Health Services in the United States, 1875–1965* (1968); and Daniel M. Fox, *Economists and Health Care: From Reform to Relativism* (1979). Competent special examinations of the leading prepaid health insurance plan are Odin W. Anderson, *Blue Cross since 1929: Accountability and the Public Trust* (1975); and Sylvia A. Law, *Blue Cross: What Went Wrong*, 2d ed. (1976).

Two excellent works cover the early phases of the movement for federal social security, including health insurance: Roy Lubove, *The Struggle for Social Security 1900–1935* (1968); and Ronald L. Numbers, *Almost Persuaded: American Physicians and Compulsory Health Insurance, 1912–1920* (1978). Later developments are examined in Daniel Hirschfield, *The Lost Reform: The Campaign for Compulsory Health Insurance in the United States from 1932 to 1943* (1970); and Ronald L. Numbers, ed., *Compulsory Health Insurance: The Continuing American Debate* (1982). The most recent phases of the movement are ably reviewed in Theodore R. Marmor and Jan S. Marmor, *The Politics of Medicare* (1970); and Robert Stevens and Rosemary Stevens, *Welfare Medicine in America: A Case Study of Medicaid* (1974). For the role of a leading life insurance firm in medicine and health, see Louis I. Dublin, *After Eighty Years: The Impact of Life Insurance on the Public Health* (1966).

The development of America's principal federal health agency is dealt with in Ralph C. Williams, *The United States Public Health Service 1798–1950* (1951); and Bess Furman, *A Profile of the United States Public Health Service 1798–1948* (1973), both of them awkwardly organized but filled with detail. A more recent, heavily pictorial account, is Fitzhugh Mullan, *Plagues and Politics: The Story of the United States Public Health Service* (1989). A short-lived early health agency is examined in Peter Bruton, "The National Board of Health, 1879–1893," Ph.D. diss. (1974). Wyndham D. Miles, *A History of the National Library of Medicine* (1982), is a thorough study. For the health-related programs of the Department of Agriculture, see Gladys L. Baker, Wayne D. Rasmussen, Vivian Wiser, and Jane M. Porter, *Century of Science: The First 100 Years of the United States Department of Agriculture* (1963). Edward D. Berkowitz, *Disabled Policy: America's Programs for the Handicapped* (1987), is a critique of poorly coordinated federal efforts in the twentieth century on behalf of the various large categories of the disabled.

Histories of medical matters in the Army include Stanhope Bayne-Jones, *The Evolution of Preventive Medicine in the United States Army, 1607–1939* (1968); and Percy M. Ashburn, *A History of the Medical Department of the United States Army* (1929). More detailed treatments are two recent volumes by Mary C. Gillett, *The Army Medical Department 1775–1818* (1981); and her, *The Army Medical Department, 1818–1865* (1987). Robert S. Henry, *The Armed Forces Institute of Pathology: Its First Century, 1862–1962* (1964), is among other things an informative history of the Army Medical Museum and of various military medical research activities. Biographies of some of the more notable Army medical figures include John M. Gibson, *Soldier in White: The Life of General George Miller Sternberg* (1958); and John M. Gibson, *Physician to the World: The Life of William C. Gorgas* (1950). There is no comprehensive history of American naval medicine.

Medical histories of the individual American wars are spotty in their coverage. For the Revolution, special treatments include Philip Cash, *Medical Men at the Siege of Boston, April 1775–April 1776* (1973); and Maurice B. Gordon, *Naval and Maritime Medicine during the American Revolution* (1978). Among the biographies, see Richard L. Blanco, *Physician of the American Revolution, Jonathan Potts* (1979). Civil War medicine is excellently treated in H. H. Cunningham, *Doctors in Gray: The Confederate Medical Service* (1958); and George W. Adams, *Doctors in Blue: The Medical History of the Union Army in the Civil War* (1952). Civilian medical support programs for the Northern armies during the Civil War are reviewed in Charles Stillé, *History of the United States Sanitary Commission* (1866), the official history; and from the perspective of modern scholarship in William Q. Maxwell, *Lincoln's*

Fifth Wheel: The Political History of the United States Sanitary Commission (1956). The medical histories of America's twentieth-century wars have, for the most part, been buried in the highly technical multi-volume official accounts. However, see J. Phinney Baxter, *Scientists against Time* (1946), an authoritative history of the World War II activities of the Office of Scientific Research and Development; and Albert E. Cowdrey, *The Medic's War* (1987), a well-written study of the Korean War.

INDEX